The Cyt

Drug Interaction Principles for Medical Practice

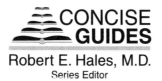

CONCISE
GUIDES

Robert E. Hales, M.D.
Series Editor

CONCISE GUIDE TO

The Cytochrome P450 System

Drug Interaction Principles for Medical Practice

Kelly L. Cozza, M.D.
Scott C. Armstrong, M.D.

With Chapter Contributions by

Michael A. Cole, M.D.
Jessica R. Oesterheld, M.D.

American **P**sychiatric Publishing, Inc.

Washington, DC
London, England

Copyright © 2001 American Psychiatric Publishing, Inc.
04   03   02   4   3
ALL RIGHTS RESERVED
Manufactured in the United States of America on acid-free paper

American Psychiatric Publishing, Inc.
1400 K Street, NW
Washington, DC 20005
www.appi.org

Library of Congress Cataloging-in-Publication Data
Cozza, Kelly L.
    Concise guide to the cytochrome P450 system : drug interaction principles for medical
practice / Kelly L. Cozza, Scott C. Armstrong ; with chapter contributions by
Michael A. Cole, Jessica R. Oesterheld.
        p. ; cm. – (Concise guides)
    Includes bibliographical references and index.
    ISBN 1-58562-000-9 (alk. paper)
    1. Cytochrome P-450—Handbooks, manual, etc. 2. Drug—Metabolism—Handbooks,
manuals, etc. 3. Psychopharmacology—Handbooks, manuals, etc. 4. Drug
interactions—Handbooks, manuals, etc. I. Armstong, Scott C. II. Cole, Michael A.,
M.D. III. Oesterheld, Jessica R. IV. Title. V. Concise guides (American Psychiatric Press)
    [DNLM: 1. Cytochrome P-450—metabolism—Handbooks. 2. Psychotropic
Drugs—pharmacokinetics—Handbooks. 3. Drug Interactions—Handbooks. 4. Mental
Disorders—drug therapy—Handbooks. QV 39 C882c 2001]
QP671.C83 C69 2001
615´.788—dc21

                                                                                00-046471

British Library Cataloguing in Publication Data
A CIP record is available from the British Library.

Thanks to my husband, Steve, and my children, Vincent and Cecilia, for their love and understanding during the preparation of this book. A special thanks to all of my mentors from or affiliated with Walter Reed Army Medical Center.
—*KLC*

Thanks to my wife, JoAnn, who was patient and understanding of my time away while I researched and wrote this book, and to my three children, Joey, Katie, and Caleb.
—*SCA*

We dedicate this book to our patients, and to all clinicians who may use this book to help in caring for them. They are the reason we are doing this work.

CONTENTS

PART I
Introduction to the P450 System
and Basic Pharmacology

PART II
P450 Enzymes

PART III
P450 Considerations by
Medical Specialty

LIST OF TABLES

CONTRIBUTORS

Scott C. Armstrong, M.D.
Co-Medical Director, Center for Geriatric Psychiatry,
Tuality Forest Grove Hospital, Forest Grove, Oregon; and
Fellow, Academy of Psychosomatic Medicine

Michael A. Cole, M.D.
Staff, Walter Reed Army Medical Center, Washington, D.C.; and
Clinical Instructor, Uniformed Services University of the Health
Sciences, Bethesda, Maryland

Kelly L. Cozza, M.D.
Psychiatrist, Infectious Disease Service, Department of Medicine,
Walter Reed Army Medical Center, Washington, D.C.;
Assistant Professor, Department of Psychiatry, Uniformed
Services University of the Health Sciences, Bethesda, Maryland;
and Fellow, Academy of Psychosomatic Medicine

Jessica R. Oesterheld, M.D.
Associate Professor, Department of Psychiatry, University of South
Dakota School of Medicine, Sioux Falls, South Dakota

INTRODUCTION

to the Concise Guides Series

The Concise Guides Series from American Psychiatric Publishing, Inc., provides, in an accessible format, practical information for psychiatrists, psychiatry residents, and medical students working in a variety of treatment settings, such as inpatient psychiatry units, outpatient clinics, consultation-liaison services, and private office settings. The Concise Guides are meant to complement the more detailed information to be found in lengthier psychiatry texts.

The Concise Guides address topics of special concern to psychiatrists in clinical practice. The books in this series contain a detailed table of contents, along with an index, tables, figures, and other charts for easy access. The books are designed to fit into a lab coat pocket or jacket pocket, which makes them a convenient source of information. References have been limited to those most relevant to the material presented.

Robert E. Hales, M.D., M.B.A.
Series Editor, Concise Guides

PREFACE

The development of this Concise Guide began as a necessity. As consecutive program directors for a busy military, tertiary-care, hospital-based consultation-liaison psychiatry service and fellowship program, we found ourselves being called on to evaluate drug interactions, as well as to teach about them to our students and colleagues. When we began to put this topic together, it was only to gain a better understanding of drug-drug interactions ourselves. It was frustrating to read articles and case reports that did not include full explanations of the topic. Some of the literature was contradictory, and the names of the enzymes seemed to change before our eyes. What began as a few tables, carried around in our pockets, became a formal lecture series. These P450 workshops grew from bedside and local grand rounds to pharmacy and therapeutics committee round tables.

Eventually, the topic followed us when we left the military. In time, we came to believe that our knowledge of the topic had evolved into something more than that of the average clinician. Our handout had grown from 8 pages to more than 50 pages by 1998. We find that software packages are typically designed for the pharmacist and do not have the depth necessary for a clinical psychiatrist to make quick, yet well-informed decisions. We realized that a book was needed. However, there is one potential major limitation to a book: it may be somewhat outdated by the time of publication. The reader is cautioned that new drugs will have been introduced and older drugs will have new interactions described after the publication of this guide. During the preparation of this book, cisapride, mibefradil, and grepafloxacin were voluntarily removed from the

United States market because of their P450-mediated interactions. This guide has been designed to enable psychiatrists to develop individualized tables and references for their own practices.

Because of length restrictions in the Concise Guides, references in each chapter of this book support both the text and the tables. Most references are cited within the text; those that are not cited are included because they support data in the tables.

The aforementioned limitations aside, we hope that readers will use this guide to quickly determine and even to anticipate drug interactions. It is designed to be used in the clinic and at the bedside as a tool for making rational and informed decisions when prescribing. We believe that this guide will provide clinicians with the information they need to prescribe appropriately in this age of polypharmacy.

PART I

Introduction to the P450 System and Basic Pharmacology

INTRODUCTION TO P450 AND TO THIS CONCISE GUIDE

An understanding of drug interactions has become essential to the practice of medicine. The increasing pharmacopoeia, coupled with prolonged human life spans, makes polypharmacy commonplace. The need for a thorough understanding of the P450 system (in this guide, we use the term *P450* rather than *cytochrome P450* or *CYP450*) became apparent in the 1980s, when the combination of terfenadine and antibiotics or of selective serotonin reuptake inhibitors and tricyclic antidepressants resulted in arrhythmias and sudden death. Despite burgeoning data and clear manufacturer warnings, patients are still at risk for drug-drug interactions.

■ WHY IS IT IMPORTANT TO UNDERSTAND THE P450 SYSTEM?

The P450 enzymes are where a large number, if not the majority, of the clinically relevant pharmacokinetic drug-drug interactions occur. Drug interactions have become an important preventable iatrogenic complication. In the United States, as many as 3% of hospitalizations per year are due to drug-drug interactions (Jankel and Fitterman 1993). The amount spent on these hospitalizations exceeds $1 billion (Johnson and Bootman 1995). In one large study involving Medicaid patients ($n = 315,084$), the risk of hospitalization greatly increased when patients were prescribed azole antifungals (odds ratio, 3.43) or rifamycins (odds ratio, 8.07), two drug classes that have significant P450 drug-drug interaction profiles

(Hamilton et al. 1998). In addition, a study by the Institute of Medicine in the United States indicated that adverse medication reactions—including drug-drug interactions—account for up to 7,000 deaths annually in the United States (Kohn et al. 2000). Clearly, drug-drug interactions are a problem that clinicians need to appreciate. These data also seem to be an underrepresentation of the situation. Many interactions are not reported by patients to physicians or by physicians to monitoring agencies. Ineffective drug therapy and annoying side effects are often not followed up thoroughly.

■ WHAT IS THE P450 SYSTEM AND WHY DOES IT EXIST?

P450 enzymes may have originated from a common ancestral gene or protein in plants and animals billions of years ago. Initially, they may have helped maintain cell membrane integrity through their contribution to steroid metabolism. As animals evolved and ate plants to survive, plants that developed toxins survived. Animals then needed to be able to detoxify these chemicals, and thus an elaborate detoxification system, the P450 system, developed (Jefferson and Greist 1996).

P450 enzymes are oxidase systems. These enzymes oxidize endogenous and exogenous compounds and usually render them less active (see Chapters 2 and 3), preparing them for elimination from the body. The P450 system's primary role is to metabolize endogenous compounds such as steroids and neuropeptides. A secondary role, especially for enzymes in the gastrointestinal system, is to detoxify ingested chemicals. These exogenous, or xenobiotic, chemicals are compounds in foods, medicines, smoke, and anything else that is an ingested organic molecule. The P450 system did not initially develop to help humans metabolize drugs. Drugs are one of the "toxins" in the modern human environment (others include pesticides and organic solvents), and P450's role in metabolizing drugs is a relatively recent phenomenon in human history. P450 enzymes are indiscriminate in their activity; they will metabolize an ancient food chemical as readily as they will metabolize a modern drug. P450 enzymes are also multifunctional; each enzyme is capable of metabolizing many different compounds.

More than 40 individual P450 enzymes have been identified in humans. However, many of these enzymes play minor roles in drug metabolism. Six enzymes are responsible for more than 90% of human drug oxidation: 1A2, 3A4, 2C9, 2C19, 2D6, and 2E1 (Guengerich 1997). These six enzymes are discussed throughout this Concise Guide.

Genetic variability exists in human P450 enzymes. It is speculated that the variety of and differences in human P450 genotypes are the result of isolated populations' evolving different abilities to survive local stressors—in this case, to metabolize indigenous organic compounds (see Chapter 3). As ethnic isolation has become replaced by diversity within the modern world, the genotypic variation of P450 has become less predictable. The evolutionary advantage of genetic variability has disappeared for modern humans. Variability in drug response is now sometimes considered an obstacle rather than an advantage.

Gender may also play a role in the development of the P450 system. However, it is difficult to establish gender differences, because these differences can be obscured by the large interindividual variation in P450 quantity and efficiency (e.g., 3A efficiency varies 3- to 13.9-fold [de Wildt et al. 1999] in the general population). Furthermore, to uncover P450-based gender distinctions in in vivo studies, one must factor out gender-based differences. It is difficult and costly to control factors related to weight and volume of distribution, ethnicity and polymorphism, smoking and alcohol consumption, obesity, age, cotherapy (including hormone replacement therapy and oral contraceptives), and gender differences in pharmacodynamics. It has been theorized that 3A4 activity may be about 20% greater in women (Harris et al. 1995). 1A2 activity and non-cytochrome phase II glucuronidation may be greater in men than in women (Tanaka 1999). Although the data on P450 gender differences are not complete, some clinically useful information is emerging on this topic. Increased serum levels of clozapine (Jerling et al. 1997) and olanzapine (Callaghan et al. 1999) in women may be a result of P450 gender differences in metabolism.

Finally, there is variability in the P450 system over the life cycle. Women's developmental changes, from menstruation to pregnancy to menopause, may affect gene expression and phenotypic variability. P450 enzymes generally "come on line," or become active, during fetal development and in the first 3–4 months of infancy (Oesterheld 1998). Of all P450 enzymes, 3A demonstrates the most variability over the life cycle. Fetuses and newborns have primarily 3A7, but the enzyme levels decrease after birth and are replaced by 3A4 (de Wildt et al. 1999) (Table 1–1). Other P450 enzymes have low activity initially, and that activity increases quickly to adult levels in the first year of life—but detailed information on the enzymes is incomplete (Hakkola et al. 1998). Latency-aged children are thought to have more efficient enzymes, accounting for their higher dose requirements of P450-metabolized drugs (e.g., tricyclic antidepressants or carbamazepine). These changes in dosing requirements disappear after puberty; teenagers past puberty require doses similar to those required by adults.

TABLE 1–1. Perinatal activity of P450 enzymes

1st trimester	2nd trimester	Birth surge	1st few weeks after birth	3–4 months after birth
3A7	3A5	2D6	3A4	1A2
1A1	2E1	2C9		
	2D6,[a] 2Cs[a]	2C19		

[a]Variably expressed.

■ HOW TO USE THIS GUIDE

This Concise Guide is designed to be a practical pocket guide—a reference at the bedside, on rounds, or in the office. The text is divided into several sections.

Part I, "Introduction to the P450 System and Basic Pharmacology," is a succinct review of pharmacology, written with psychiatrists in mind. We recommend reading this section first and then returning to particular chapters in the section as needed when consulting later chapters or reviewing other current literature.

Part II, "P450 Enzymes," contains pertinent tables, short reviews, and carefully chosen clinical and research illustrations for each P450 enzyme (such as 2D6 or 3A4). Particular emphasis is placed on psychotropic drugs and their metabolism. This section will perhaps be frequently consulted once the reader is familiar with the nomenclature and the pertinent literature to date. We and many of our mentors carry lists such as these to refer to when we cannot remember where in the system a particular drug is metabolized or which drug inhibits or induces metabolism at which enzyme site. These chapters conclude with case vignettes, to provide an opportunity for study and to better illustrate drug interactions in clinical practice.

Part III, "P450 Considerations by Medical Specialty," is unique to this text. The drugs commonly used in nonpsychiatric medicine that have clinically significant P450-related drug interactions are arranged by specialty (and listed in tables), with pertinent clinical and research data to support and clarify the issues. We recommend a quick review *before* seeing any inpatient or outpatient with concomitant medical-surgical problems. Some of the data in this section's tables are the same as in Part II, so each part can stand alone.

We have gathered the tables from Parts I and II into a pullout pocket guide to provide a quick and convenient reference to the P540 tables.

Appendix A, "Guidelines," consists of suggestions about prescribing multiple drugs and monitoring for drug interactions. Recommendations are made regarding which psychotropics, at the time of publication, are safest when multiple drugs are prescribed.

In Appendix B, "How to Retrieve and Review the Literature," we share the approach we developed in culling the enormous and sometimes confusing amount of information available in this area. The reader will be better able to find and evaluate new data in the current literature. We hope that this section will help clinicians to become more drug-interaction expert in their own fields, as they identify useful references and develop practice-specific drug lists of their own.

Finally, we remind the reader that drugs interact in many ways. An adverse drug reaction may occur without involvement of the P450 system. Nevertheless, hepatic and gut wall P450 interactions are in the majority. We do not review all types of interactions here (absorption, protein-binding, renal excretion and elimination, and pharmacodynamic interactions are excluded), and we refer the reader elsewhere for information on those specific interactions.

■ REFERENCES

Callaghan JT, Bergstrom RF, Ptak LR, et al: Olanzapine: pharmacokinetic and pharmacodynamic profile. Clin Pharmacokinet 37:177–193, 1999

de Wildt SN, Kearns GL, Leeder JS, et al: Glucuronidation in humans: pharmacogenetic and developmental aspects. Clin Pharmacokinet 36:439–452, 1999

Guengerich FP: Role of cytochrome P450 enzymes in drug-drug interactions. Adv Pharmacol 43:7–35, 1997

Hakkola J, Tanaka E, Pelkonen O: Developmental expression of cytochrome P450 enzymes in human liver. Pharmacol Toxicol 82:209–217, 1998

Hamilton RA, Briceland LL, Andritz MH: Frequency of hospitalization after exposure to known drug-drug interactions in a Medicaid population. Pharmacotherapy 18:1112–1120, 1998

Harris RZ, Benet LZ, Schwartz JB: Gender effects in pharmacokinetics and pharmacodynamics. Drugs 50:222–239, 1995

Jankel CA, Fitterman LK: Epidemiology of drug-drug interactions as a cause of hospital admissions. Drug Saf 9:51–59, 1993

Jefferson JW, Greist JH: Brussels sprouts and psychopharmacology: understanding the cytochrome P450 enzyme system. Psychiatr Clin North Am: Annual of Drug Therapy 3:205–222, 1996

Jerling M, Merle Y, Mentre F, et al: Population pharmacokinetics of clozapine evaluated with the nonparametric maximum likelihood method. Br
J Clin Pharmacol 44:447–453, 1997

Johnson JA, Bootman JL: Drug-related morbidity and mortality: a cost-of-
illness model. Arch Intern Med 155:1949–1956, 1995

Kohn L, Corrigan J, Donaldson M (eds): To Err Is Human: Building a Safer
Health System. Washington, DC, National Academy Press, 2000

Oesterheld JR: A review of developmental aspects of cytochrome P450.
J Child Adolesc Psychopharmacol 8:161–174, 1998

Tanaka E: Gender-related differences in pharmacokinetics and their clinical
significance. J Clin Pharm Ther 24:339–346, 1999

2

BASIC PHARMACOLOGY

Drug interactions reflect a shift in drug activity or effect in the body as a result of another drug's presence or activity. Drug interactions are usually considered either pharmacodynamic or pharmacokinetic. In this chapter, we outline pharmacodynamic and pharmacokinetic principles. Special emphasis is placed on pharmacokinetics and the mechanisms of metabolism because the mixed function oxygenase or monooxidase microsomal system of metabolism is the P450 system.

■ DRUG INTERACTIONS DEFINED

Pharmacodynamic Interactions

Pharmacodynamic interactions are interactions due to one drug's influence on another drug's effect at the latter's intended receptor site or end organ. These interactions or alterations in drug function are not due to a change in absorption, distribution, metabolism, or elimination. When two drugs act at a receptor site in the brain, causing a combined, typically unwanted effect or negating a wanted effect, a pharmacodynamic interaction is said to have occurred. The potentially dangerous monoamine oxidase inhibitor and tricyclic antidepressant serotonin syndrome is an example of a pharmacodynamic interaction.

Pharmacokinetic Interactions

Pharmacokinetic interactions are interactions due to one drug's effect on the movement of another drug through the body. These interactions are alterations in the way the body would normally metabolize a drug in its effort to eliminate it. Pharmacokinetic interactions may result in delayed onset of effect, decreased or increased effect, toxicity, or altered excretion, and they directly affect the concentration of drug that reaches the target site. Pharmacokinetic interactions encompass alterations in absorption, distribution, metabolism, or excretion.

Absorption interaction: An alteration due to one drug's effect on another drug's route of entry into the body. Most absorption interactions occur in the gut; some examples of these interactions are altered gastric pH, food coadministration, mechanical blockade or chelation, and loss of gut flora.

Distribution interaction: An alteration in how a drug travels throughout the body; typically a result of alterations in protein binding in plasma. Drug effect is directly related to the amount of free drug available to the target site. More or less drug is available if another drug displaces the protein-bound fraction of a drug. Warfarin is an example of a drug that is sensitive to protein-binding displacement by many other drugs.

Metabolism interaction: An alteration in the biotransformation of a compound into active drug or excretable inactive compounds; usually results in a change in drug concentration due to a slowing or "backing up" of or an increase in enzymatic metabolism. In this Concise Guide, metabolism is covered in great depth.

Excretion interaction: An alteration in the ability to eliminate an unaltered drug or metabolite from the body. An example of this type of interaction is the effect of sodium concentration or diuretics on lithium retention by the kidneys.

■ METABOLISM

Drugs are usually lipophilic, which allows them to enter their site of action at target organs or tissues via cell membranes and exert their effect. Lipophilic compounds are difficult to eliminate from the body. Metabolism, or biotransformation of these compounds into more polar, inactive metabolites, is necessary and is generally an enzymatic process.

Biotransformation occurs throughout the body, with the greatest concentration of activity in the liver and the gut wall. At the cellular level, biotransformation occurs in the endoplasmic reticulum. With many drugs, there is a *first-pass effect* as the drug crosses the gut wall and again as the drug passes through the liver, before reaching the systemic circulation and its target sites. Most drugs lose functional activity during the "first pass" as the body begins the process of preparing the drug for elimination. This first-pass effect can limit the oral availability of drugs and is a factor in determining whether a drug should be administered parenterally or orally. P450 metabolism occurs in the gut wall, with 3A4 making up 70% of intestinal P450 (DeVane 1998). The kidneys, lungs, and skin also have significant metabolic activity, and any cell with endoplasmic reticulum has the capacity for some metabolic reactions.

Phase I Metabolism

Phase I reactions add or expose a functional group on a compound or drug through oxidative reactions such as *N*-dealkylation, *O*-dealkylation, hydroxylation, *N*-oxidation, *S*-oxidation, or deamination (see Table 2–1). The resulting compounds may then lose all pharmacological activity when they are ready for reactions to form highly water soluble conjugates and for elimination by means of phase II metabolism. In actuality, many drugs are not metabolized in this linear fashion, and some may undergo conjugation reactions of phase II before phase I, or these reactions may occur simultaneously. Some drugs do not lose pharmacological activity at all; instead, their activity is enhanced. The cytochrome P450 monooxygenase system is a phase I system.

Cytochrome P450 Monooxidase System

More than 200 P450 enzymes exist in nature, and a collection of at least 40 enzymes is found in humans. Six enzymes comprise about

TABLE 2–1. Major drug biotransformation reactions

Reaction	Phase I	Examples
I. Oxidative reactions		
N-Dealkylation	$RNHCH_3 \longrightarrow RNH_2 + CH_2O$	Imipramine, diazepam, codeine, erythromycin, morphine, tamoxifen, theophylline
O-Dealkylation	$ROCH_3 \longrightarrow ROH + CH_2O$	Codeine, indomethacin, dextromethorphan
Aliphatic hydroxylation	$RCH_2CH_3 \longrightarrow R\overset{\displaystyle OH}{C}HCH_3$	Tolbutamide, ibuprofen, pentobarbital, meprobamate, cyclosporine, midazolam
Aromatic hydroxylation		Phenytoin, phenobarbital, propranolol, phenylbutazone, ethinyl estradiol

TABLE 2–1. Major drug biotransformation reactions *(continued)*

Reaction	Phase I		Examples
I. Oxidative reactions			
N-Oxidation	$RNH_2 \longrightarrow RNHOH$		Chlorpheniramine, dapsone
	$\begin{matrix} R_1 \\ \diagdown \\ NH \\ \diagup \\ R_2 \end{matrix} \longrightarrow \begin{matrix} R_1 \\ \diagdown \\ N{-}OH \\ \diagup \\ R_2 \end{matrix}$		Guanethidine, quinidine, acetaminophen
S-Oxidation	$\begin{matrix} R_1 \\ \diagdown \\ S \\ \diagup \\ R_2 \end{matrix} \longrightarrow \begin{matrix} R_1 \\ \diagdown \\ S{=}O \\ \diagup \\ R_2 \end{matrix}$		Cimetidine, chlorpromazine, thioridazine
Deamination	$\underset{\underset{NH_2}{\mid}}{RCHCH_3} \rightarrow R-\underset{\underset{NH_2}{\mid}}{\overset{\overset{OH}{\mid}}{C}}-CH_3 \rightarrow R-\overset{\overset{O}{\parallel}}{C}-CH_3 + NH_2$		Diazepam, amphetamine

TABLE 2–1. Major drug biotransformation reactions *(continued)*

Reaction	Examples
II. Hydrolysis reactions	
$\underset{R_1COR_2}{\overset{O}{\parallel}} \longrightarrow R_1COOH + R_2OH$	Procaine, aspirin, clofibrate
$\underset{R_1CNR_2}{\overset{O}{\parallel}} \longrightarrow R_1COOH + R_2NH_2$	Lidocaine, procainamide, indomethacin
III. Conjugation reactions Phase II	
Glucuronidation UDP-glucuronic acid	Acetaminophen, morphine, diazepam

TABLE 2–1. **Major drug biotransformation reactions** *(continued)*

Reaction		Examples
III. Conjugation reactions	**Phase II**	
Sulfation	ROH + 3'-phosphoadenosine-5'-phosphosulfate (PAPS) → R—O—S—OH ($=O$, $=O$) + 3'-phosphoadenosine-5'-phosphate	Acetaminophen, steroids, methyldopa
Acetylation	CoAS—C($=O$)—CH₃ (acetyl-coenzyme A) + RNH₂ → RNH—C($=O$)—CH₃ + CoA-SH	Sulfonamides, isoniazid, dapsone, clonazepam

Source. Reprinted from Benet LZ, Kroetz DL, Sheiner LB: "Pharmacokinetics: The Dynamics of Drug Absorption, Distribution and Elimination," in *Goodman and Gilman's The Pharmacological Basis of Therapeutics*, 9th Edition. New York, McGraw-Hill, 1996, p. 13. With permission of the McGraw-Hill Companies.

90% of all P450 enzymes—1A2, 3A4, 2C9, 2C19, 2D6, and 2E1—
and all play an important role in xenobiotic oxidative metabolism.
These enzymes are on the smooth endoplasmic reticulum of hepatocytes and the luminal epithelium of the small intestine. These
heme-containing proteins are closely associated with nicotinamide
adenine dinucleotide phosphate (reduced form) (NADPH) cytochrome P450 reductase, which donates or is the source of the elec-
trons needed for oxidation (Benet et al. 1996). (For details on the
enzymatic reactions, see Table 2–1 and the references at the end of
this chapter.)

The P450 enzymes contain red-pigmented heme, and when
bound to carbon monoxide they absorb light at a wavelength of
450 nanometers. In the term *cytochrome P450, cyto* stands for
microsomal vesicles, P for *pigmented,* and *450* for *450 nanometers.* Each enzyme is encoded by one particular gene—one gene,
one protein. The enzymes are grouped into families and subfamilies according to the similarity of their amino acid sequences. Enzymes in the same family are homologous for 40%–55% of amino
acid sequences, and enzymes within the same subfamily are homologous for more than 55%. (See Table 2–2 for more on P450 nomenclature.)

Until the early 1990s, it was standard to label a family using a
roman numeral; an enzyme might be labeled *CYPIID6.* Today, Ar-
abic numerals are used; the same enzyme is now labeled *CYP2D6.*
In addition, the system that is the focus of this book is referred to in
several ways, including *cytochrome P450 system, CYP450 system,*
and *P450 system.* For brevity, we use *P450 system* throughout. Individual enzymes are designated several ways in the literature;
a particular enzyme might be labeled *cytochrome P450 2D6,
CYP2D6,* or *2D6.* In this book, we use the shortest forms, labeling
individual P450 enzymes *2D6* or *3A4,* for example. Finally, the
P450 enzymes are often called *isoenzymes* or *isozymes* in the literature, but these terms are misnomers because they refer to enzymes
that catalyze one reaction. To avoid confusion, the term *enzymes* is
used throughout this text.

TABLE 2–2.   **P450 nomenclature**

Category	Addition(s) to *P450*	Examples
Family	Arabic numeral	P450 1, P450 2
Subfamily	Arabic numeral + uppercase letter	P450 1A, P450 2D
Single gene or protein	Arabic numeral + uppercase letter + Arabic numeral	P450 1A2, P450 2D6

Amine Oxidase System

The amine oxidase system is also considered a part of phase I, but it is not the P450 system. This group includes monoamine oxidases (MAOs), which have been studied in relation to depression and Parkinson's disease. Strolin and Tipton (1998) provided a thorough review of what is known about non-P450 phase I metabolism.

Phase II Metabolism

In phase II or conjugation reactions, water-soluble molecules are added to a drug, usually making an inactive, easily excretable compound. Covalent linkages are made between the drug and glucuronic acid, sulfate, acetate, amino acids, and/or glutathione (Benet et al. 1996).

Phase II enzymes have not been as well studied, because recent research focus has been on the P450 or phase I enzymes. Phase I enzymes were the first to come to researchers' attention because these enzymes are more apt to produce active or toxic metabolites when they oxidize, by "taking away" methyl, alkyl, or hydroxyl groups. The vast majority of clinically important drug interactions involve P450. Nevertheless, the attention paid to phase II enzymes has increased, and it has become clear that this system has great impact on metabolic drug interactions as well. Conjugation occurs with many chemical groups, the best studied of which include amino acids, acetyl groups, ester groups, glucuronic acid, glutathione, methyl groups, and sulfate groups. What follows is an overview of three of the best-studied phase II enzymatic processes.

Glucuronidation

The most abundant phase II enzymes belong to the family of uridine 5′-diphosphate glucuronosyltransferases (UGTs). This family is a major detoxification system and the liver is the main site of glucuronidation, with the kidney having activity as well (McGurk et al. 1998). Ten UGTs have been identified in humans (de Wildt et al. 1999). These UGTs are involved in the biotransformation of many drugs, including acetaminophen, antipsychotics (e.g., clozapine, olanzapine, and quetiapine), amines (tricyclic antidepressants and antihistamines), many benzodiazepines, bupropion, morphine, nonsteroidal anti-inflammatory drugs, and zidovudine (Hawes 1998; Patel et al. 1995). UGTs also conjugate endogenous compounds, such as bilirubin, thyroid, and some steroid hormones. Chloramphenicol, a drug conjugated by UGTs, is known to produce a severe toxic reaction in the neonate, and this reaction is believed to be due to lack of development of one or more UGTs. The specifics of the 10 isoforms have not been fully elucidated, and therefore obtaining clinically useful information is not entirely possible. Although several of the isoforms have been identified with probes and inhibitors in vitro, in vivo studies are lagging behind P450 research because specific substrate probes or inhibitors for most isoforms are unclear and the isoforms have overlapping functions. See Chapter 3, Table 3–1, for more on UGT inhibition, induction, and substrates.

The view that glucuronidation leads to biologically inactive compounds is generally correct. However, some compounds made by UGTs can lead to adverse drug reactions and/or drug hypersensitivity (Burchell and Coughtrie 1997). The process of glucuronidation creates a "new" chemical, which may stimulate the immune system to respond to the glucuronidated compound adversely. Additionally, it has been shown that when morphine is metabolized by UGTs, an active analgesic, morphine-6-glucuronide, is produced (Kroemer and Klotz 1992). Finally, UGTs are also a "recycling" system, with some compounds being conjugated and then unconjugated, ultimately slowing clearance of the compound.

Methylation

Enzyme subfamilies that conjugate through methylation are almost too numerous to count. It should be noted that the effects of *S*-adenosylmethionine (SAMe, or "sammy") (which is used to treat many illnesses, including depression) may be related to methylation enzymes, because SAMe is a methyl donor compound (Bottiglieri and Hyland 1994). Three of the better-studied and more interesting methyltransferases are catechol *O*-methyltransferase (COMT), histamine *N*-methyltransferase (HNMT), and thiopurine methyltransferase.

Catechol *O*-methyltransferase. The best appreciated of the methyltransferases, COMT has been known for more than 70 years (Kopin 1994). COMT is one of two means by which catecholamines are metabolized, the other being MAOs (a non-P450 phase I system). COMTs also metabolize steroid catechols. COMTs are located in virtually all regions, the two most important of which may be the brain and the liver. There are two main forms of COMT: membrane-bound COMT and soluble COMT (Ellingson et al. 1999), and genetic polymorphisms have been noted (Kuchel 1994). Many studies have examined the genetic diversity of COMT as a factor in illness, including breast cancer, hypertension, bipolar disorder, and schizophrenia.

Selective and reversible inhibition of COMT was developed as a strategy for enhancing dopamine availability in patients with Parkinson's disease (Goldstein and Lieberman 1992). Tolcapone and entacapone are COMT-inhibiting drugs, but how they inhibit COMT is unclear.

Histamine *N*-methyltransferase. HNMT metabolizes histamine by adding a methyl group to histamine; then MAO further catabolizes the methylhistamine. HNMT is located in many regions, particularly the liver and the kidney (De Santi et al. 1998). Its gene is located on chromosome 2, and HNMT has genetic polymorphic variability, but the clinical significance of the polymorphisms are currently unclear (Preuss et al. 1998) (see "Pharmacogenetics" in Chapter 3). A common group of inhibitors, the 4-aminoquinolones (e.g., chloroquine and hydroxychloroquine), are believed to be inhibitors of HNMT, and this inhibition may account for their usefulness in treating rheumatoid arthritis, systemic lupus erythematosus (Cumming et al. 1990), and other inflammatory disorders. Another group of inhibitors of HNMTs are the steroidal neuromuscular relaxants, such as pancuronium and vecuronium. Inhibition of HNMT may explain instances of flushing and hypotension with the use of these drugs (Futo et al. 1990).

Thiopurine methyltransferase.   Thiopurine methyltransferase is best known for its rare polymorphic character. In fact, thiopurine methyltransferase's routine phenotyping in patients with leukemia who require drugs such as 6-mercaptopurine is perhaps the first use of phenotype testing to enter general practice (Weinshilboum et al. 1999). For further details, see "Pharmacogenetics" in Chapter 3 and Chapter 14, "Oncology."

Sulfation

Sulfation is the transfer of a sulfate group from 3′-phosphoadenosine 5′-phosphosulfate (PAPS) to a substrate. This reaction is catalyzed by a family of sulfotransferase enzymes. Sulfation is PAPS dependent in that PAPS can easily be "used up" in human liver in 2 minutes (Klaassen and Boles 1997), although more can quickly be made. The major sulfation enzymes have been identified, and they are polymorphic (Dooley 1998), but the full significance of this finding is unclear. Sulfation is involved in many primary and secondary pathways of endogenous and exogenous compounds, including steroid hormones, catecholamines, phenolic agents, and therapeutic drugs. A major step in troglitazone's metabolism is sulfation (Loi et al. 1999). Environmental influences are known to occur, and one of the more interesting of these influences is the apparent inhibition of sulfotransferases by components in coffee and tea (Coughtrie et al. 1998).

■ SUMMARY

In summary, drug interactions occur for many reasons. Pharmacokinetic interactions are due to an alteration in drug absorption, distribution, metabolism, or elimination. Most drug interactions are due to alterations in enzymatic processes of phase I and phase II metabolism. Interestingly, an understanding of phase I and II metabolism alone does not explain why there is so much variability in patient response to drugs. Much of this variability is due to alterations in the P450 system through environmental and genetic influences described in Chapter 3.

■ REFERENCES

Benet LZ, Kroetz DL, Sheiner LB: Pharmacokinetics: the dynamics of drug absorption, distribution and elimination, in Goodman and Gilman's The Pharmacological Basis of Therapeutics, 9th Edition. New York, McGraw-Hill, 1996, pp 3–27

Bottiglieri T, Hyland K: S-Adenosylmethionine levels in psychiatric and neurological disorders: a review. Acta Neurol Scand Suppl 154:19–26, 1994

Burchell B, Coughtrie MW: Genetic and environmental factors associated with variation of human xenobiotic glucuronidation and sulfation. Environ Health Perspect 105 (suppl 4):739–747, 1997

Coughtrie MW, Sharp S, Maxwell K, et al: Biology and function of the reversible sulfation pathway catalysed by human sulfotransferases and sulfatases. Chem Biol Interact 109:3–27, 1998

Cumming P, Reiner PB, Vincent SR: Inhibition of rat brain histamine-N-methyltransferase by 9-amino-1,2,3,4-tetrahydroacridine (THA). Biochem Pharmacol 40:1345–1350, 1990

De Santi C, Donatelli P, Giulianotti PC, et al: Interindividual variability of histamine N-methyltransferase in the human liver and kidney. Xenobiotica 28:571–577, 1998

DeVane CL: Principles of pharmacokinetics and pharmacodynamics, in The American Psychiatric Press Textbook of Psychopharmacology, 2nd Edition. Edited by Schatzberg AF, Nemeroff CB. Washington, DC, American Psychiatric Press, 1998, pp 155–169

de Wildt SN, Kearns GL, Leeder JS, et al: Glucuronidation in humans: pharmacogenetic and developmental aspects. Clin Pharmacokinet 36:439–452, 1999

Dooley TP: Cloning of the human phenol sulfotransferase gene family: three genes implicated in the metabolism of catecholamines, thyroid hormones and drugs. Chem Biol Interact 109:29–41, 1998

24

Ellingson T, Duppempudi S, Greenberg BD, et al: Determination of differential activities of soluble and membrane-bound catechol-O-methyltransferase in tissues and erythrocytes. J Chromatogr B Biomed Sci Appl 729:347–353, 1999

Futo J, Kupferberg JP, Moss J: Inhibition of histamine N-methyltransferase (HMNT) in vitro by neuromuscular relaxants. Biochem Pharmacol 39:415–420, 1990

Goldstein M, Lieberman A: The role of the regulatory enzymes of catecholamine synthesis in Parkinson's disease. Neurology 42:8–12, 41–48, 1992

Hawes EM: N+-glucuronidation, a common pathway in human metabolism of drugs with a tertiary amine group. Drug Metab Dispos 26:830–837, 1998

Klaassen CD, Boles JW: Sulfation and sulfotransferases 5: the importance of 3′-phosphoadenosine 5′-phosphosulfate (PAPS) in the regulation of sulfation. FASEB J 11:404–418, 1997

Kopin IJ: Monoamine oxidase and catecholamine metabolism. J Neural Transm Suppl 41:57–67, 1994

Kroemer HK, Klotz U: Glucuronidation of drugs: a re-evaluation of the pharmacological significance of the conjugates and modulating factors. Clin Pharmacokinet 23:292–310, 1992

Kuchel O: Clinical implications of genetic and acquired defects in catecholamine synthesis and metabolism. Clin Invest Med 17:354–373, 1994

Loi CM, Young M, Randinitis E, et al: Clinical pharmacokinetics of troglitazone. Clin Pharmacokinet 37:91–104, 1999

McGurk KA, Brierley CH, Burchell B: Drug glucuronidation by human renal UDP-glucuronyltransferases. Biochem Pharmacol 55:1005–1012, 1998

Patel M, Tang BK, Kalow W: (S)oxazepam glucuronidation is inhibited by ketoprofen and other substrates of UGT2B7. Pharmacogenetics 5:43–49, 1995

Preuss CV, Wood TC, Szumlanski CL, et al: Human histamine N-methyltransferase pharmacogenetics: common genetic polymorphisms that alter activity. Mol Pharmacol 53:708–717, 1998

Strolin BM, Tipton KF: Monoamine oxidases and related amine oxidases as phase I enzymes in the metabolism of xenobiotics. J Neural Transm Suppl 52:149–171, 1998

Weinshilboum RM, Otterness DM, Szumlanski CL: Methylation pharmacogenetics: catechol-O-methyltransferase, thiopurine methyltransferase, and histamine N-methyltransferase. Annu Rev Pharmacol Toxicol 39:19–52, 1999

3

METABOLIC VARIABILITY: INHIBITION, INDUCTION, AND PHARMACOGENETICS

Drug response varies greatly across groups and individuals. This variability is due to many pharmacological factors. In phase I and phase II metabolism, this variability may be a reflection of enzyme inhibition, enzyme induction, and/or genetic differences.

■ INHIBITION

Drugs metabolized at a common human enzyme will at times be competing or sharing metabolic sites within the P450 system in the liver and gut. A drug's affinity for an enzyme is called its *inhibitory potential* or *Ki*. Drugs with little affinity for an enzyme have a high Ki and probably will not bind. Drugs with a low Ki, or great affinity for enzyme binding, are very likely to bind and may compete with drugs for the same site. When drugs are coadministered, the drug with the greater affinity (lower Ki) will competitively inhibit the binding of the drug with lower affinity (high Ki) (Owen and Nemeroff 1998). Some drugs bind to an enzyme and inhibit its activity without needing the enzyme for their own metabolism. Some drugs may be both substrates of an enzyme (may require that enzyme for metabolism) and inhibitors of the same enzyme. Drugs that inhibit an enzyme may slow down the enzyme's activity or block the activity needed for metabolism of other drugs there, which will result in increased levels of any drug dependent on that enzyme for biotransformation. This inhibition leads to prolonged pharmacological effect and may result in drug toxicity. Inhibition is immediate in its effect, and when treatment with the offending drug is discontinued, the enzyme quickly returns to normal function. Symptoms caused by drug-drug inhibition have a rapid onset and disappear quickly.

The P450 system is greatly affected by competitive inhibition. Ketoconazole has a low Ki, or a high affinity for enzyme binding at 3A4. When coadministered with terfenadine, this drug prevented the metabolism of the parent compound of terfenadine, leading to increased serum levels of toxic terfenadine, which caused arrhythmias. Without coadministration of a potent inhibitor, terfenadine is rapidly metabolized at 3A4 to its nontoxic but pharmacodynamically active compound fexofenadine. Each human P450 enzyme is fully discussed in the chapters that follow, with tables of inhibitors provided.

Phase II metabolism is also affected by inhibition, particularly the inhibition of uridine 5′-diphosphate glucuronosyltransferases (UGTs). Oxazepam's conjugation was found to be inhibited by a variety of nonsteroidal anti-inflammatory drugs, which are conjugated by UGTs as well as oxidized by 2E1 (Patel et al. 1995). Zidovudine's metabolism has been shown to be inhibited by naproxen and probenecid (Veal and Back 1995). Cimetidine and other histamine, subtype 2 (H$_2$), receptor blockers—often known as "pan-inhibitors" of P450 enzymes—do not appear to inhibit UGTs (Irshaid and Abu-Khalaf 1992). The inhibitors of UGTs appear to vie with the other substrates to be conjugated by the UGTs. Listed in Table 3–1 are the known inhibitors of UGTs.

■ INDUCTION

Some xenobiotics, both drugs and environmental substances such as cigarette smoke, increase the synthesis of P450 proteins, actually increasing the number of sites available for biotransformation. When more sites are available, more compound is metabolized at a time. This induction process may lead to decreases in the amount of parent drug administered and increases in the number of metabolites produced. An inducer may cause the level of a coadministered drug

TABLE 3–1.   **Phase II uridine 5′-diphosphate glucuronosyltransferase (UGT) substrates, inhibitors, and inducers**

Substrates[a]	Inhibitors	Inducers
Acetaminophen	NSAIDs	Clofibrate
Antihistamines (H$_1$)	Probenecid	Dexamethasone
Antipsychotics		
Benzodiazepines		
Bilirubin		
Bupropion		
Entacapone/tolcapone		
Lamotrigine		
Mianserin		
Morphine		
NSAIDs		
Steroid hormones		
Tricyclic antidepressants		
Zidovudine		

Note.   NSAID = nonsteroidal anti-inflammatory drug.
[a]Substrates are also metabolized by other phase I and II enzymes.

to decrease to below the level needed for therapeutic effect, resulting in loss of clinical efficacy. For example, coadministration of the potent inducer rifampin and methadone has led to opiate withdrawal (see Chapter 12 and "Analgesics" in Chapter 15). Drugs that require P450 metabolism for activation may become toxic if active metabolites are produced more quickly than expected. Such a phenomenon is hypothesized to occur with the induction of valproic acid: the production of toxic metabolites is increased, leading to hepatotoxicity (see Chapter 13). 3A4, 1A2, 2C9, 2C19, and 2E1 may all be induced. 2D6 does not appear to be inducible, but this concept is currently being debated; "pan-inducers" such as phenobarbital and rifampin need further study at 2D6 (Venkatakrishnan et al. 1999; von Bahr et al. 1998). Clinically significant P450 enzymes vulnerable to induction are discussed in the chapters that follow.

Phase II metabolism, particularly the UGTs (Gueraud and Paris 1998), may also be subject to induction by drugs such as the pan-inducer phenobarbital. Clofibrate and dexamethasone may also be inducers of some of the isoforms of UGTs (Jemnitz et al. 2000; Vecchini et al. 1995). The new combination protease inhibitor Kaletra (lopinavir/ritonavir) has been found to induce glucuronidation and may reduce effectiveness of other coadministered antiretroviral (HIV) drugs, such as zidovudine and abacavir, by increasing risk of viral resistance to these drugs (Abbott Laboratories, Products Division personal communication, December 2000). Kaletra may also decrease effectiveness of methadone (Abbott Laboratories, Products Division personal communication, December 2000). Evidence to date does not indicate that the rifamycins induce UGTs (Fromm et al. 1997; Reinach et al. 1999). The evolutionary significance of induction is obvious, given that UGTs are involved in the metabolism of many endogenous (steroid and thyroid) hormones. The ability to regulate hormone metabolism is necessary to maintain homeostasis. See Table 3–1 for a list of UGT substrates, inhibitors, and inducers.

■ PHARMACOGENETICS: POLYMORPHISMS

Clinicians have noted for decades that drug metabolism greatly varies across racial groups. The genetic variability (polymorphisms) of P450 is arguably the most important clinical pharmacogenetic consideration (Eichelbaum and Evert 1996). The concept of racially polymorphic enzymes makes intuitive sense. Enzymes exist in part to metabolize exogenous substances in human environments, and therefore different populations developed different enzyme capabilities, based on exposure to particular environmental stressors.

The term *genetic polymorphism* refers to the ability of individuals to metabolize drugs to differing degrees due to differences in enzyme capacity and function. Some individuals are considered *poor metabolizers* (PMs): their metabolism is slower or they are less able to biotransform a compound compared with the rest of a population. *Ultraextensive metabolizers* (UEMs), also called ultrarapid metabolizers (URMs) in older literature, require more drug than expected to achieve therapeutic effect, because of the rapidity with which their enzymes metabolize a compound. Average metabolizers, called *extensive metabolizers* (EMs) or rapid metabolizers (RMs) in older literature, may be "converted" to PMs by P450 inhibitors. Although these "converted" individuals are not genetically determined to metabolize poorly, they mimic genetic PMs and are thus "phenotypic" PMs. Most P450 and some phase II enzymes are polymorphic. See Table 3–2 for information on P450 polymorphisms.

Genetic Polymorphisms in Depth

The polymorphic variability of drug metabolism was empirically recognized before the P450 system was well understood. Slow and rapid acetylators of isoniazid were recognized in the 1950s. Glucose-6-phosphate dehydrogenase deficiency leading to hemolytic anemia was appreciated as a genetically based variation in drug metabolism. In the 1970s, Ziegler and Biggs (1977) noted that black patients had significantly higher nortriptyline levels than did other patients, and the investigators assumed there were genetic differences. These differences in nortriptyline metabolism are now believed to result from genetic polymorphisms related to 2D6, 2C9, and/or 2C19.

Knowledge of genetic polymorphisms of P450 has exploded since the late 1990s, when it became possible to test genetically on a clinical level. Table 3–2 is a current guide to the genetic polymorphisms of P450. With new polymorphisms being identified by researchers almost daily, this list is sure to grow.

Genotypic or phenotypic testing of P450 enzymes is being incorporated into some practice protocols (Crespi and Miller 1999; Tanaka and Breimer 1997). For example, activity of 2D6, which has a polymorphism that renders some people poor metabolizers for drugs that use 2D6, may be premeasured through administration of a probe drug, such as dextromethorphan. Probes are drugs that are metabolized, often exclusively, by an enzyme, resulting in a measurable and reliable metabolite. Dextromethorphan is exclusively metabolized by 2D6 to dextrophan. A patient who has no dextrophan after ingesting dextromethorphan likely lacks 2D6 activity.

TABLE 3–2. P450 polymorphisms

CYP450	Polymorphisms	Type(s)	Phenotype substrate probes[a]	Drugs that warrant caution for PMs
2D6	Yes	PM, EM, UEM	Debrisoquin, dextromethorphan, sparteine	Antiarrhythmics, codeine, tramadol
3A4	Possible	Unknown	Cyclosporine, erythromycin, lidocaine, midazolam	Unknown
1A2	Probable	Unknown	Caffeine, theophylline	Unknown
2C9	Yes	PM, EM	Naproxen, phenytoin, tolbutamide	S-warfarin
2C19	Yes	PM, EM	Proguanil	Cyclophosphamide, ifosfamide
2E1	Yes	Unclear	Chlorzoxazone	Anesthestic agents

Note. EM=extensive metabolizer; PM=poor metabolizer; UEM=ultraextensive metabolizer.
[a]Probes are metabolized by one identified P450 enzyme into a specific known metabolite.

Predetermining 2D6 phenotypes would help one to adequately treat patients who require codeine or tramadol. Codeine is metabolized by 2D6 to morphine (Ozdemir et al. 1996), and tramadol is essentially a pro-drug metabolized by 2D6 to the more active analgesic compound M1 (Dayer et al. 1997) (see "Analgesics" in Chapter 15). Knowing that a patient is a PM before initiation of pharmacotherapy would allow one to target treatment for better analgesia.

Another illustration of "probing" for genetic variability to guide therapy is found in cancer chemotherapy. A person who lacks thiopurine methyltransferase, a phase II conjugation enzyme (these individuals make up 0.3% of the population), may have a fatal response to normal doses of thiopurines (Keuzenkamp-Jansen et al. 1996) (see Chapter 14). Most clinicians do not routinely genotype patients. It is expected that in the future, as physicians continue to prescribe multiple drugs, increasing reliance will be placed on the use of probes or similar methods to genetically fingerprint patients (Tanaka and Breimer 1997). Such methods will become most useful in situations in which drugs either are activated by enzymes (pro-drugs; e.g., codeine [2D6] and cyclophosphamide [2C19]) or are dangerous at high levels (e.g., some antiarrhythmics [metabolized by 2D6] and S-warfarin [2C9]) (Linder and Valdes 1999).

■ REFERENCES

Crespi CL, Miller VP: The use of heterologously expressed drug metabolizing enzymes—state of the art and prospects for the future. Pharmacol Ther 84:121–131, 1999

Dayer P, Desmeules J, Collart L: Pharmacology of tramadol. Drugs 53 (suppl 2):18–24, 1997

Eichelbaum M, Evert B: Influence of pharmacogenetics on drug disposition and response. Clin Exp Pharmacol Physiol 23:983–985, 1996

Fromm MF, Eckhardt K, Li S, et al: Loss of analgesic effect of morphine due to coadministration of rifampin. Pain 72:261–267, 1997

Gueraud F, Paris A: Glucuronidation: a dual control. Gen Pharmacol 31: 683–688, 1998

Hawes EM: N+-glucuronidation, a common pathway in human metabolism of drugs with a tertiary amine group. Drug Metab Dispos 26:830–837, 1998

Irshaid Y, Abu-Khalaf M: Lack of effect of certain histamine H2-receptor blockers on the glucuronidation of 7-hydroxy-4-methylcoumarin by human liver microsomes. Pharmacol Toxicol 71:294–296, 1992

Jemnitz K, Veres Z, Monostory K, et al: Glucuronidation of thyroxine in primary monolayer cultures of rat hepatocytes: in vitro induction of UDP-glucuronosyltransferases by methylcholanthrene, clofibrate, and dexamethasone alone and in combination. Drug Metab Dispos 28:34–37, 2000

Keuzenkamp-Jansen CW, Leegwater PA, De Abreu RA, et al: Thiopurine methyltransferase: a review and a clinical pilot study. Journal of Chromatography. B, Biomedical Applications 678:15–22, 1996

Linder MW, Valdes R: Pharmacogenetics in the practice of laboratory medicine. Molecular Diagnostics 4:365–379, 1999

Owen JR, Nemeroff CB: New antidepressants and the cytochrome P450 system: focus on venlafaxine, nefazodone and mirtazapine. Depress Anxiety 7 (suppl 1):24–32, 1998

Ozdemir V, Fourie J, Busto U, et al: Pharmacokinetic changes in the elderly: do they contribute to drug abuse and dependence? Clin Pharmacokinet 31:372–385, 1996

Patel M, Tang BK, Kalow W: (S)oxazepam glucuronidation is inhibited by ketoprofen and other substrates of UGT2B7. Pharmacogenetics 5:43–49, 1995

Reinach B, de Sousa G, Dostert P, et al: Comparative effects of rifabutin and rifampicin on cytochromes P450 and UDP-glucuronosyl-transferases expression in fresh and cryopreserved human hepatocytes. Chem Biol Interact 121:37–48, 1999

Tanaka E, Breimer DD: In vivo function tests of hepatic drug-oxidizing capacity in patients with liver disease. J Clin Pharm Ther 22:237–249, 1997

Veal GJ, Back DJ: Metabolism of zidovudine. Gen Pharmacol 26:1469–1475, 1995

Vecchini F, Mace K, Magdalou J, et al: Constitutive and inducible expression of drug metabolizing enzymes in cultured human keratinocytes. Br J Dermatol 132:14–21, 1995

Venkatakrishnan K, von Moltke LL, Greenblatt DJ: Nortriptyline E-10-hydroxylation in vitro is mediated by human CYP2D6 (high affinity) and CYP3A4 (low affinity): implications for interactions with enzyme-inducing drugs. J Clin Pharmacol 39:567–577, 1999

von Bahr C, Steiner E, Koike Y, et al: Time course of enzyme induction in humans: effect of pentobarbital on nortriptyline metabolism. Clin Pharmacol Ther 64:18–26, 1998

Ziegler VE, Biggs JT: Tricyclic plasma levels: effect of age, race, sex, and smoking. JAMA 238:2167–2169, 1977

PART II

P450 Enzymes

4

2D6

2D6 is usually discussed first in reviews of the P450 system because of the historical role this enzyme played in the development of an understanding of drug interactions. In 1988, Vaughan noted very high serum levels of desipramine and nortriptyline when fluoxetine was concomitantly administered. More reports followed Vaughan's report on two cases, and by 1990 the P450 system was recognized as being responsible for this potentially dangerous interaction (von Ammon Cavanaugh 1990). In 1991, Muller et al. identified 2D6 as the enzyme that fluoxetine inhibits, and this finding was confirmed in 1992 by Skjelbo and Brosen. 2D6 became the most studied of the hepatic enzymes in the early 1990s. Since that time, however, 3A4 has overtaken 2D6 as a focus of research and clinical interest, because of the sheer magnitude of drugs affected by 3A4.

■ WHAT DOES 2D6 DO?

2D6 is involved in phase I metabolism of endogenous and exogenous compounds. Its actions include hydroxylation, demethylation, and dealkylation of compounds. 2D6's activity does not appear to change with age (Shulman and Ozdemir 1997), but it may be slightly lower in women than in men (Tanaka 1999).

■ WHERE IS 2D6?

2D6 is found in many tissues (including the brain), but it plays its role in drug metabolism in the liver. 2D6 actually makes up only

1.5% of the total P450 content in the liver, the smallest percentage with regard to the six P450 enzymes described in this text. Nevertheless, 2D6 is a very active primary or secondary participant in the metabolism of many drugs.

■ DOES 2D6 HAVE ANY POLYMORPHISMS?

Yes. Clinically, this is the most important fact to remember about this enzyme. The *2D6* gene is located on chromosome 22. It appears that up to 14% of Caucasians have a defective, autosomal recessive allele(s). People of other races appear to have this phenotype less frequently (Belpaire and Bogaert 1996; de Leon et al. 1998). Individuals homozygous for the defective allele(s) are phenotypically labeled *poor metabolizers* (PMs). Persons with normal 2D6 activity are called *extensive* or *rapid metabolizers.* In addition, 1%–3% of individuals have a third phenotype. These persons seem to have extra copies of the allele and are able to metabolize some compounds faster and more extensively. Individuals with this third phenotype are referred to as *ultraextensive metabolizers* (Eichelbaum and Evert 1996).

Polymorphisms have been noted for many years (Vesell et al. 1971). In the 1980s, 2D6 was named in relation to its probes; it was called the debrisoquin/sparteine enzyme (Eichelbaum 1986). By 1990, its polymorphic character was well recognized, and 2D6 was given its current name (Lennard 1990).

Any drug that is primarily metabolized by 2D6 and ingested by a PM will have a slowed metabolism. The PM will accumulate parent drug, usually resulting in enhanced effects. PMs usually require lower doses to achieve desired effects. However, we suspect that in many clinical situations, a patient who is not recognized as a PM cannot tolerate either the side effects or increased serum levels of a drug. These results are then assumed to be due to a drug interaction or some unknown idiosyncratic response, and treatment with the poorly metabolized drug may be abandoned. However, many drugs can be given to a 2D6 PM; the clinician need only decrease the dose. Not anticipating that patients are PMs is potentially dangerous. For example, the action of some antiarrhythmics depends on 2D6 metabolism. If a patient lacks 2D6 activity, severe toxicity may occur if an antiarrhythmic such as encainide is prescribed (Funck-Brentano et al. 1992).

A drug may be less effective for a PM of 2D6 as well, particularly if the drug needs to be activated at 2D6. Codeine and tramadol are pro-drugs metabolized by 2D6 to more active analgesic compounds (see "Analgesics" in Chapter 15 for more details). A clinician might repeatedly increase the dose of the drug in an attempt to achieve the desired effect, with poor results—leaving the patient and the clinician frustrated. Occasionally, a clinician labels a patient as "drug seeking," when in fact the patient is unable to metabolize prodrug to active drug at 2D6.

Risperidone is metabolized by 2D6 to its active 9-OH metabolite. In PMs at 2D6, the drug is primarily metabolized by 3A4. Anecdotal evidence suggests that PMs at 2D6 have a poorer tolerance of side effects and higher drug levels, even though the alternate 3A4 route is available (Bork et al. 1999).

There is a way to determine whether a patient is a PM of 2D6, yet this method is rarely practiced clinically. One can probe for the phenotype by giving a drug primarily metabolized by 2D6 and looking for the specific 2D6 metabolites. Dextromethorphan, the over-the-counter cough remedy, is one such drug; debrisoquin and sparteine are two others. After the patient is administered a fixed single dose of dextromethorphan, the clinician can determine whether 2D6 activity is present by measuring the active metabolite specific to 2D6, dextrophan (created by 2D6's O-demethylation of dextromethorphan), in the blood or urine (Schadel et al. 1995).

■ ARE THERE DRUGS THAT INHIBIT 2D6 ACTIVITY?

Yes. The selective serotonin reuptake inhibitors (SSRIs), particularly fluoxetine and paroxetine, are the best-known inhibitors of this enzyme (Greenblatt et al. 1998).

Selective Serotonin Reuptake Inhibitors

Fluoxetine, paroxetine, and even sertraline (at high doses; e.g., 200 mg/day) strongly inhibit 2D6 (Richelson 1997). These drugs can increase levels of tricyclic antidepressants and antipsychotics, can inhibit the ability of codeine and tramadol to control pain, and may increase serum antiarrhythmic levels. Recently, the U.S. FDA and the drug manufacturer issued a warning that 2D6 inhibitors and thioridazine should not be coadministered (Food and Drug Administration 2000).

Typically, inhibition of P450 enzymes is competitive and dependent on the relative affinities of the compounds for the enzyme. Because the inhibition is competitive, once an inhibitor is introduced, inhibition is immediate. Removing the inhibitor will quickly negate the inhibition, and enzyme activity will return to normal levels within a few days, the time dependent on the half-life of the inhibitor. One exception to this quick reversal, however, is the reversal of fluoxetine. Fluoxetine (and its active metabolite, norfluoxetine) has a long half-life, approximately 5–14 days. When fluoxetine is removed, a 4- to 8-week washout period elapses before enzyme activity returns to normal.

Cimetidine

Cimetidine appears to be a potent and indiscriminate inhibitor of several enzymes, including 2D6, 3A4, and 1A2 (Martinez et al. 1999). Other histamine, subtype 2 (H_2), receptor blockers, such as ranitidine, are not as problematic (see Chapter 11). Cimetidine has been found to increase paroxetine serum levels by 50% (Greb et al. 1989). Although paroxetine itself is a potent inhibitor of 2D6, cimetidine's affinity for 2D6 is greater (lower inhibitory potential [Ki]).

■ ARE THERE DRUGS THAT INDUCE 2D6 ACTIVITY?

Probably not. Using 10-hydroxylation of nortriptyline as a probe for 2D6 activity, von Bahr et al. (1998) found that pentobarbital appears to induce other P450 enzymes but not 2D6. However, there is some evidence that phenobarbital and smoking may decrease serum concentrations of 2D6 substrates. It is unclear whether this decrease is due to induction or to other mechanisms.

■ REFERENCES

Belpaire FM, Bogaert MG: Cytochrome P450: genetic polymorphism and drug interactions. Acta Clin Belg 51:254–260, 1996

Bork JA, Rogers T, Wedlund PJ, et al: A pilot study on risperidone metabolism: the roles of cytochromes P450 2D6 and 3A. J Clin Psychiatry 60:469–476, 1999

Caccia S: Metabolism of the new antidepressants: an overview of the pharmacological and pharmacokinetic implications. Clin Pharmacokinet 34:281–302, 1998

de Leon J, Barnhill J, Rogers T, et al: Pilot study of cytochrome P450-2D6 genotype in a psychiatric hospital. Am J Psychiatry 155:1278–1280, 1998

Eichelbaum M: Polymorphic oxidation of debrisoquine and sparteine. Prog Clin Biol Res 214:157–167, 1986

Eichelbaum M, Evert B: Influence of pharmacogenetics on drug disposition and response. Clin Exp Pharmacol Physiol 23:983–985, 1996

Ereshefsky L: Pharmacokinetics and drug interactions: update for newer antipsychotics. J Clin Psychiatry 57 (suppl 11):12–25, 1997

Food and Drug Administration: Novartis Pharmaceuticals' warning of Mellaril (thioridazine) (FDA Talk Paper T2000-34ME). Rockville, MD, National Press Office, July 25, 2000 [www.fda.gov/opacom/hpwhats.html]

Funck-Brentano C, Thomas G, Jacqz-Aigrain E, et al: Polymorphism of dextromethorphan metabolism: relationships between phenotype, genotype and response to the administration of encainide in humans. J Pharmacol Exp Ther 263:780–786, 1992

Greb WH, Buscher G, Dierdorf HD, et al: The effect of liver enzyme inhibition by cimetidine and enzyme induction by phenobarbitone on the pharmacokinetics of paroxetine. Acta Psychiatr Scand Suppl 350:95–98, 1989

Greenblatt DJ, von Moltke LL, Harmatz JS, et al: Drug interactions with newer antidepressants: role of human cytochromes P450. J Clin Psychiatry 59 (suppl 15):19–27, 1998

Lennard MS: Genetic polymorphism of sparteine/debrisoquine oxidation: a reappraisal. Pharmacol Toxicol 67:273–283, 1990

Martinez C, Albet C, Agundez JA, et al: Comparative in vitro and in vivo inhibition of cytochrome P450 CYP1A2, CYP2D6, and CYP3A by H2-receptor antagonists. Clin Pharmacol Ther 65:369–376, 1999

Muller N, Brockmoller J, Roots I: Extremely long plasma half-life of amitriptyline in a woman with the cytochrome P450IID6 29/29-kilobase wild-type allele—a slowly reversible interaction with fluoxetine. Ther Drug Monit 13:533–536, 1991

Richelson E: Pharmacokinetic drug interactions of the new antidepressants: a review of the effects on the metabolism of other drugs. Mayo Clin Proc 72:835–847, 1997

Schadel M, Wu D, Otton SV, et al: Pharmacokinetics of dextromethorphan and metabolites in humans: influence of the CYP2D6 phenotype and quinidine inhibition. J Clin Psychopharmacol 15:263–269, 1995

Shulman RW, Ozdemir V: Psychotropic medications and cytochrome P450 2D6: pharmacologic considerations in the elderly. Can J Psychiatry 42 (suppl 1):4S–9S, 1997

Skjelbo E, Brosen K: Inhibitors of imipramine metabolism by human liver microsomes. Br J Clin Pharmacol 34:256–261, 1992

Tanaka E: Gender-related differences in pharmacokinetics and their clinical significance. J Clin Pharm Ther 24:339–346, 1999

Vaughan DA: Interaction of fluoxetine with tricyclic antidepressants (letter). Am J Psychiatry 145:1478, 1988

Vesell ES, Passananti GT, Greene FE, et al: Genetic control of drug levels and of the induction of drug-metabolizing enzymes in man: individual variability in the extent of allopurinol and nortriptyline inhibition of drug metabolism. Ann N Y Acad Sci 179:752–773, 1971

von Ammon Cavanaugh S: Drug-drug interactions of fluoxetine with tricyclics. Psychosomatics 31:273–276, 1990

von Bahr C, Steiner E, Koike Y, et al: Time course of enzyme induction in humans: effect of pentobarbital on nortriptyline metabolism. Clin Pharmacol Ther 64:18–26, 1998

■ STUDY CASES

Vignette 1

A 30-year-old Caucasian woman with schizoaffective disorder stopped taking thioridazine. She had been taking 200 mg/day with good clinical efficacy and few side effects for 5 years. She was hospitalized 1 month after stopping thioridazine therapy, because of increasing agitation and depressive symptoms. Initially, she consented to recommencing thioridazine therapy, and the dose was titrated back to 200 mg/day within 1 week. After 1 week, she agreed to try an antidepressant, and she was prescribed fluoxetine 20 mg/day. Five days after starting fluoxetine therapy, the patient developed extrapyramidal symptoms.

Comment

2D6 inhibition: Although there have been reports of treatment with fluoxetine alone causing extrapyramidal symptoms, it seems likely that the symptoms in this case were caused by the increased serum levels of thioridazine that resulted from fluoxetine's 2D6 inhibition. Thioridazine, as well as other typical neuroleptics, is metabolized by 2D6.

References

Blake BC, Rose RL, Mailman RB, et al: Metabolism of thioridazine by microsomal monooxygenases: relative role of P450 and flavin-containing monooxygenases. Xenobiotica 25:377–393, 1995

Kurlan R: Acute parkinsonism induced by the combination of a serotonin reuptake inhibitor and a neuroleptic in adults with Tourette's disorder. Mov Disord 13:178–179, 1998

Vignette 2

A 17-year-old Caucasian boy with bipolar disorder, a seizure disorder, and mild mental retardation was taking haloperidol (5 mg/day), valproic acid (1,750 mg/day), benztropine (4 mg/day), gabapentin (300 mg/day), and buspirone (10 mg/day). Paroxetine therapy (20 mg/day) was started because of depressive symptoms. On the eighth day of paroxetine therapy, the patient reported that he had a dry mouth and nausea; was disoriented to time, disorganized, forgetful, and lethargic; and had slurred speech. Vital signs were unremarkable, and he exhibited no extrapyramidal symptoms. Pupils were dilated and sluggish to respond. Treatment with paroxetine, haloperidol, benztropine, and valproic acid was discontinued. Serum levels were as follows: valproic acid, 119 µg/mL (previous levels, 103–105 µg/mL); haloperidol, 2.9 ng/mL (therapeutic range, 5–12 ng/mL); and gabapentin, 4.1 µg/mL (therapeutic range, 4–16 µg/mL). His serum benztropine level was 35.9 ng/mL; levels greater than 25 ng/mL are considered toxic. Two days after discontinuation of the medications, the patient reported feeling better. He resumed treatment with haloperidol and valproic acid without incident.

Comment

2D6 inhibition: Benztropine is an older drug whose metabolism has not been well characterized. Seven cases in the literature indicate that SSRIs may interact with benztropine because of inhibition of benztropine metabolism. Because fluoxetine, paroxetine, and sertraline inhibit 2D6, it is hypothesized that benztropine is at least in part metabolized by 2D6. We suggest that in this case, paroxetine's inhibition increased serum benztropine levels, causing a mild anticholinergic delirium.

References

Armstrong SC, Schweitzer SM: Delirium associated with paroxetine and benztropine combination. Am J Psychiatry 154:581–582, 1997

Byerly MJ, Christensen RC, Evans OL: Delirium associated with a combination of sertraline, haloperidol and benztropine. Am J Psychiatry 153:965–966, 1996

Roth A, Akyol S, Nelson JC: Delirium associated with a combination of a neuroleptic, an SSRI and benztropine. J Clin Psychiatry 55:492–495, 1994

Vignette 3

A 36-year-old African American woman was taking paroxetine (20 mg/day) for depression. She tried tramadol and oxycodone preparations for pain and found them largely unhelpful. At a pain clinic, use of mexiletine (an antiarrhythmic that is also used for chronic pain disorders and is dependent on 2D6 for metabolism) was considered. Because of concerns that the patient might not metabolize mexiletine adequately, the patient's psychiatrist strongly urged the team to try an alternative drug.

Comment

PM of 2D6: The psychiatrist surmised that the reason the patient did not have a good response to codeine or tramadol was that she was a phenotypic PM of 2D6, either because of the paroxetine or because of her genetic expression. Tramadol and oxycodone are pro-drugs that are activated by metabolism of the parent compound at 2D6. Although the psychiatrist did not determine this patient's 2D6 genotype, she believed caution was necessary before use of an antiarrhythmic that is also metabolized by 2D6 was undertaken.

References

Hedenmalm K, Sundgren M, Granberg K, et al: Urinary excretion of codeine, ethylmorphine, and their metabolites: relation to the CYP2D6 activity. Ther Drug Monit 19:643–649, 1997

Labbe L, Turgeon J: Clinical pharmacokinetics of mexiletine. Clin Pharmacokinet 37:361–384, 1999

Paar WD, Poche S, Gerloff J, et al: Polymorphic CYP2D6 mediates O-demethylation of the opioid analgesic tramadol. Eur J Clin Pharmacol 53:235–239, 1997

■ DRUGS METABOLIZED BY 2D6

Antidepressants	Antipsychotics	Other drugs	
Tricyclic antidepressants[1]	*Antipsychotics*		*Cardiovascular drugs*[2]
Amitriptyline	Clozapine[3]		Diltiazem
Clomipramine	Haloperidol[2]		Encainide
Desipramine	Perphenazine[2]		Flecainide
Imipramine	Quetiapine[2]		Mexiletine
Nortriptyline	Risperidone[2]		Nifedipine
	Thioridazine[2]		Nisoldipine
Other antidepressants			Propafenone
Fluoxetine[2]			Propranolol[6]
Maprotiline	*Analgesics*		
Mirtazapine[2]	Codeine[4]		
Paroxetine[2]	Hydrocodone		
Sertraline	Methadone[2]		
Trazodone[2]	Oxycodone		
Venlafaxine[2]	Tramadol[5]		
	Miscellaneous drugs		
	Benztropine[2]		
	Delavirdine[2]		
	Dextromethorphan[7]		
	Donepezil[2]		
	Ondansetron[2]		
	Tacrine[2]		
	Tamoxifen[2]		

[1]Tricyclic antidepressants (TCAs) use several enzymes for metabolism. The secondary tricyclics are preferentially metabolized by 2D6, the tertiary tricyclics by 3A4. TCAs are also metabolized by 1A2, 2C9, and 2C19.
[2]Metabolized by other P450 enzymes.
[3]2D6 is a minor pathway; 3A4 and 1A2 are more prominent.
[4]Metabolized by 2D6 to morphine.
[5]Metabolized to a more active pain-relieving compound, M1.
[6]β-Blockers are partly or primarily metabolized by 2D6.
[7]Used as a probe for 2D6 activity.

■ INHIBITORS OF 2D6

Antidepressants	Antipsychotics	Other inhibitors
Fluoxetine[a]	Fluphenazine	**Cimetidine**[a]
Fluvoxamine	Haloperidol[c]	Lansoprazole
Norfluoxetine[a]	Perphenazine	Lopinavir/ritonavir[3]
Paroxetine[a]	Thioridazine[b,c]	Methylphenidate
Sertraline[1]		**Quinidine**[2,a]
		Ritonavir[a]
		Terbinafine
		Valproic acid
		Yohimbine

[1]Sertraline's inhibition seems to be dose specific, with higher doses resulting in more potent inhibition than lower doses.
[2]Quinidine's inhibition is stereospecific. Its isomer, quinine, does not inhibit.
[3]Kaletra inhibits 2D6 in vitro. In vivo studies pending at time of publication.

[a]Potent (bold type).
[b]Moderate.
[c]Mild.

5

3A4

3A4 enzymes are involved in the metabolism of numerous drugs, accounting for the majority of the cytochrome enzymes in the liver and the gut wall. Twenty-five to 30% of P450 enzymes in the liver are 3A4, and more than half of the gut wall's P450 enzymes are 3A4 (Zhang et al. 1999). These closely related enzymes have been named 3A3, 3A4, 3A5, and 3A7 in humans. 3A7 is expressed in utero and is replaced by 3A3, 3A4, and 3A5 soon after birth. 3A3, 3A4, and 3A5 have very similar amino acid sequences and functions and are therefore usually labeled as one enzyme, 3A4.

■ WHAT DOES 3A4 DO?

3A4 is involved in phase I metabolism of endogenous and exogenous compounds. This activity includes hydroxylation, demethylation, and dealkylation of substrates. 3A4 is an important enzyme in the metabolism of endogenous steroids through 6β-hydroxylation. Children and young adults seem to have more 3A4 function than do adults, and this enzyme may be more active in women than in men. More study on gender differences is needed (Tanaka 1999).

Because 3A4 accounts for so much of P450 activity, it should not be a surprise that many drugs are metabolized by 3A4. Indeed, the list of medications metabolized by 3A4 is constantly growing, and 3A4 may account for more than half of all human liver drug oxidation (Guengerich 1999).

■ WHERE IS 3A4?

As noted earlier, 3A4 is located primarily in the liver and gut wall. 3A3 is present particularly in the gut wall, 3A4 in hepatocytes, and 3A5 in the kidney. The enzyme is also located in other tissues throughout the body.

■ DOES 3A4 HAVE ANY POLYMORPHISMS?

No, none of any clinical significance (Westlind et al. 1999). Expression varies from individual to individual, being 10- to 30-fold greater in some persons (Ketter et al. 1995). The gene or genes for the enzyme are located on chromosome 7. There seem to be some differences with age, as noted earlier. Because 3A4 accounts for so much of P450 activity, it is not clear whether the decrease in activity with age is specific to 3A4 or to all P450 enzymes.

■ ARE THERE DRUGS THAT INHIBIT 3A4 ACTIVITY?

Yes. Clinically, this is the most important fact to remember about this system. Several classes of drugs, and a chemical found in grapefruit and its juice (Fuhr 1998), potently inhibit 3A4. With so many drugs metabolized by 3A4, one would expect many serious consequences of inhibition of 3A4 activity, particularly in the case of drugs that are highly dependent on 3A4 activity and that have narrow therapeutic windows or margins of safety.

Despite their notoriety for inhibiting P450 enzymes, selective serotonin reuptake inhibitors (SSRIs) are not the worst inhibitors of 3A4. SSRIs, except for citalopram (which is a mild inhibitor), are only moderate inhibitors of 3A4. The only psychotropic drug that is a potent inhibitor of 3A4 is nefazodone, a non-SSRI antidepressant (Owen and Nemeroff 1998).

Nonpsychotropics that are potent inhibitors include azole antifungals, macrolide antibiotics, and antiretrovirals (Albengres et al. 1998; Barry et al. 1997; Caspi 1998; Eagling et al. 1997; Tseng and

Foisy 1997; Von Rosensteil and Adam 1995). Many psychotropic drugs are partially to fully metabolized by 3A4 (Ketter et al. 1995), and when these drugs are combined with any of the potent 3A4 inhibitors, the inhibitors may wreak havoc on drug levels and cause significant toxicity and adverse side effects. For example, two deaths in 1997 were associated with concomitant use of clarithromycin and pimozide (Desta et al. 1999; Food and Drug Administration 1996). Clarithromycin, a commonly used macrolide that potently inhibits 3A4, had been added to pimozide, which is metabolized by 3A4. High serum levels of pimozide can cause significant and life-threatening prolongation of the QTc interval. Most manufacturers now state that use of any inhibitor of 3A4 during pimozide therapy is contraindicated.

Before prescribing psychotropics, physicians must determine what drugs the patient is taking. Additionally, patient education may prevent other physicians from unknowingly prescribing combinations that may cause problems. Reminding patients who are on drugs with narrow therapeutic windows to call their primary care provider before taking any newly prescribed drug may be a lifesaving practice.

Inhibition of 3A4: Historical Issues

In the late 1990s, several 3A4-related casualties occurred, and drugs were removed from the United States market by manufacturers.

Nonsedating Antihistamines

In 1997, terfenadine was voluntarily withdrawn from the United States market by its manufacturer. Astemizole was withdrawn in 1999. These histamine, subtype 1 (H_1), receptor antagonists were pro-drugs that required 3A4 for metabolism to their active ingredients. However, the parent compounds were toxic to the cardiac conduction system and at high levels caused supraventricular tachycardia and/or torsades de pointes. Significant interactions occurred when inhibitors of 3A4 were prescribed with these drugs. Terfenadine is no longer available, but its nontoxic active metabolite, fexofenadine, is. Fexofenadine is excreted by the kidneys unchanged and, even at high serum levels, is not associated with cardiac toxicity (see "Allergy Drugs" in Chapter 11).

Mibefradil

Mibefradil, a calcium-channel blocker, was voluntarily removed from the United States market in 1998 because of its toxicity as a potent inhibitor of 3A4 and 2D6. The drug also inhibited 1A2. Although warnings were updated as interactions and potential interactions became apparent, physicians continued to prescribe it. Just before the manufacturer's withdrawal, the Food and Drug Administration (1998) published a Talk Paper that included a long list of drugs that could have dangerous effects when administered with mibefradil. Because many other calcium-channel blockers are available, the manufacturer removed it from distribution.

Cisapride

Cisapride was removed from the United States market in July 2000. This agent is metabolized by 3A4 and can have serious cardiac effects. A total of 341 cases of cardiac arrhythmia have been reported, including 80 fatalities. Eighty-five percent of these interactions involved 3A4 inhibitors or drugs that could cause arrhythmia (Food and Drug Administration 2000). Study of the use of low-dose cisapride to reduce SSRI-induced nausea did not reveal any adverse cardiac events (Bergeron and Plier 1994).

Inhibition of 3A4: Current Issues

Triazolobenzodiazepines

Triazolobenzodiazepines—alprazolam, midazolam, estazolam, and triazolam—are substrates of 3A4. Caution is warranted when these drugs are used with most SSRIs, nefazodone, and other inhibitors of 3A4. The manufacturer of nefazodone has recommended a 50% reduction in dose of alprazolam and a 75% reduction in dose of triazolam when they are coadministered with nefazodone (Serzone package insert 1995). Case reports and reports of small controlled studies have indicated enhanced effects (including severe sedation and delirium) when triazolobenzodiazepines are used with inhibitors of 3A4, such as ritonavir (von Moltke et al. 1998), erythromycin (Tokinaga et al. 1996), and even diltiazem, a moderate inhibitor (Kosuge et al. 1997).

Nonbenzodiazepine Hypnotics

The nonbenzodiazepine hypnotics zolpidem and zaleplon are metabolized by 3A4. Enhanced effects are expected when these drugs are used with 3A4 inhibitors. However, there are no published reports of excessive sedation with coadministration of 3A4 inhibitors and either zolpidem or zaleplon. Package inserts warn of potential interactions between zolpidem or zaleplon and 3A4 inhibitors (see, for example, the Norvir [ritonavir] package insert [1996], and later in this chapter, we present a case in which ritonavir enhanced the effects of zolpidem).

Selective Serotonin Reuptake Inhibitors

Although they are only moderate inhibitors of 3A4, SSRIs may be problematic. Administration of fluoxetine with a calcium-channel blocker has resulted in enhanced cardiac side effects (Azaz-Livshits and Danenberg 1997). Although nifedipine and diltiazem are 3A4 inhibitors, their affinity for 3A4 is weaker than the affinities of fluoxetine and paroxetine.

Buspirone

Buspirone is mainly metabolized by 3A4. Enhanced effects of the drug (mainly sedation) have been reported with coadministration of buspirone and either erythromycin or itraconazole, the latter two drugs increasing buspirone levels 5–13 times (Kivisto et al. 1997). One would expect the same result with coadministration of buspirone and other 3A4 inhibitors.

Grapefruit Juice

Grapefruit juice is also a potent inhibitor at 3A4. A chemical unique to grapefruit inhibits 3A4 in the gut wall (Edwards et al. 1996). Drinking just 8 ounces of grapefruit juice has been associated with significant increases in levels of calcium-channel blockers (Fuhr 1998). Excessive drowsiness was reported when grapefruit juice was given with triazolam (Hukkinen 1995). Kivisto et al. (1997) found that grapefruit juice increased plasma concentrations of cisapride in healthy volunteers and warned of the risk of this combination in patients at risk for arrhythmia. We expect that serum levels of clozapine, tricyclic antidepressants, and other antidepressants are affected by grapefruit juice as well (no studies have been reported). Grapefruit juice may also inhibit 1A2 by a different mechanism, broadening its interaction spectrum. In addition, grapefruit juice may also worsen side effects of oral contraceptives, because the juice can increase peak levels of ethinyl estradiol by 137% (Weber et al. 1996).

Drug Sparing and Augmentation

Some authors have advocated using grapefruit juice as a sparing agent (to reduce the amount spent on expensive drugs such as cyclosporine or some protease inhibitors). This strategy should be avoided because grapefruit juice concentrations are not constant, even within the same brand. Timing grapefruit juice ingestion (i.e., planning juice ingestion a few hours before or after 3A4-dependent medications are taken) can be disastrous. We instruct our patients to avoid grapefruit juice, and one of us (SCA) has had it removed from the menu at a hospital, to avoid serious interactions.

The use of 3A4 inhibitors to enhance effects of drugs or increase levels, and therefore decrease the amount spent on expensive drugs, deserves some comment. In 1995, Keogh et al. reported that concomitant use of ketoconazole and cyclosporine reduced the dose of the latter drug by 80% and reduced the amount spent on that drug per patient by an average of $5,200. A subsequent report indicated that long-term use of ketoconazole may have risks, such as reduction of bone mineralization (L. W. Moore et al. 1996). Drug-sparing strategies must be initiated cautiously (see "Immunosuppressants" in Chapter 15).

Psychiatrists have engaged in enhancement of drug effects for some time. Cimetidine was used for years to augment the effects of clozapine, until potential toxicity was recognized (Szymanski et al. 1991). Cimetidine is an inhibitor of 2D6, 3A4, and 1A2 and can increase clozapine levels. Likewise, some clinicians have used SSRIs to augment clozapine's effects, and some physicians have proposed using an SSRI to decrease the amount spent on clozapine (Armstrong and Stephans 1997). Maintaining safe serum levels of clozapine with these drug combinations is difficult, and at times the risk of very high levels of clozapine may outweigh any gains. One series indicated a 43% increase in serum clozapine or norclozapine levels when clozapine was administered with fluoxetine, paroxetine, or sertraline (Centorrino et al. 1996). Fluvoxamine (which strongly inhibits both 3A4 and 1A2, the two main enzymes needed for metabolism of clozapine) is the worst offender. Wetzel et al. (1998) demonstrated a *threefold* increase in the serum level and half-life of clozapine or norclozapine with the addition of just 50 mg of fluvoxamine per day. Interestingly, the coadministration of fluvoxamine and clozapine has been found, in a well-monitored setting, to be both safe and economically beneficial in schizophrenic patients requiring clozapine (Lu et al. 2000).

■ ARE THERE DRUGS THAT INDUCE 3A4 ACTIVITY?

Yes. The best-known inducer of 3A4 is carbamazepine. For years it was known that carbamazepine induced its own metabolism. Neurologists and psychiatrists recognized that after initiation of carbamazepine therapy, an upward dose adjustment would be necessary within 4–8 weeks to maintain stable carbamazepine levels. The mechanism is now known: carbamazepine induces 3A4, and the drug is also metabolized by 3A4 (Levy 1995). Carbamazepine induces not only 3A4 but also phase II conjugation enzymes (Ketter et al. 1999).

Oxcarbazepine, a drug developed to have fewer drug interactions and adverse side effects than carbamazepine, does induce 3A4 and can induce the metabolism of oral contraceptives, rendering them less effective (Fattore et al. 1999). Other antiepileptics are in-

54

ducers as well, including phenytoin, phenobarbital, and primidone (Anderson 1998).

There is evidence that the antitubercular drugs rifampin and rifabutin (Strayhorn et al. 1997), the nonnucleoside reverse transcriptase inhibitors nevirapine and efavirenz (Barry et al. 1997; Tseng and Foisy 1997), troglitazone (Caspi 1997), and dexamethasone and prednisone (Pichard et al. 1992) all induce 3A4. Modafinil, a central nervous system stimulant, has been shown to induce its own metabolism at high doses, and 3A4 is the enzyme induced (Provigil package insert 1999). Finally, there is growing evidence that the herbal supplement St. John's wort may induce 3A4 (L.B. Moore et al. 2000; Roby et al. 2000), causing transplant rejection by decreasing cyclosporine levels (Barone et al. 2000; Karliova et al. 2000; Ruschitzka et al. 2000), and a decline in digoxin levels (Johne et al. 1999).

Ritonavir, although a potent inhibitor of 3A4, *induces* 3A4 metabolism after a few weeks. It has been found to increase the metabolism of meperidine, resulting in increased levels of the neurotoxic metabolite normeperidine, and to reduce the area under the curve (AUC) and maximal drug concentration (C_{max}) of ethinyl estradiol (EE) (Ouellet et al. 1998; Piscitelli et al. 2000). There are no reports to date of ritonavir compromising the effectiveness of coadministered protease inhibitors that rely on 3A4 metabolism, and, in fact, it has recently been introduced as a combination protease inhibitor with lopinavir (see Chapter 12).

■ REFERENCES

Albengres E, LeLouet H, Tillement JP: Systemic antifungal agents: drug interactions of clinical significance. Drug Saf 18:83–97, 1998

Anderson GD: A mechanistic approach to antiepileptic drug interactions. Ann Pharmacother 32:554–563, 1998

Armstrong SC, Stephans JR: Blood clozapine levels elevated by fluvoxamine: potential for side effects and lower clozapine dosage (letter). J Clin Psychiatry 58:499, 1997

Azaz-Livshits TL, Danenberg HD: Tachycardia, orthostatic hypotension and profound weakness due to concomitant use of fluoxetine and nifedipine. Pharmacopsychiatry 30:274–275, 1997

Barone GW, Gurley BJ, Ketel BL, et al: Drug interaction between St. John's wort and cyclosporine. Ann Pharmacother 34:1013–1016, 2000

Barry M, Gibbons S, Mulchay F: Protease inhibitors in patients with HIV disease: clinically important pharmacokinetic considerations. Clin Pharmacokinet 32:194–209, 1997

Bergeron R, Plier P: Cisapride for the treatment of nausea produced by selective serotonin inhibitors. Am J Psychiatry 151:1084–1086, 1994

Caspi A: Troglitazone. Pharmacy and Therapeutics 22:198–205, 1997

Caspi A: Therapeutic advantages of the newer fluoroquinolones. Pharmacy and Therapeutics 23:18–28, 1998

Centorrino F, Baldessarini RJ, Frankenburg FR, et al: Serum levels of clozapine and norclozapine in patients treated with selective serotonin reuptake inhibitors. Am J Psychiatry 153: 820–822, 1996

Desta Z, Kerbusch T, Flockhart DA: Effect of clarithromycin on the pharmacokinetics and pharmacodynamics of pimozide in healthy poor and extensive metabolizers of cytochrome P450 2D6 (CYP2D6). Clin Pharmacol Ther 65:10–20, 1999

Eagling VA, Back DJ, Barry MG: Differential inhibition of cytochrome P450 isoforms by the protease inhibitors, ritonavir, saquinavir and indinavir. Br J Clin Pharmacol 44:190–194, 1997

Edwards DJ, Bellevue FH 3rd, Woster PM: Identification of 6′,7′-dihydroxybergamottin, a cytochrome P450 inhibitor, in grapefruit juice. Drug Metab Dispos 24:1287–1290, 1996

Fattore C, Cipolla G, Gatti G, et al: Induction of ethinylestradiol and levonorgestrel metabolism by oxcarbazepine in healthy women. Epilepsia 40:783–787, 1999

Food and Drug Administration: Report of pimozide and macrolide antibiotic interaction. FDA Medical Bulletin 26:3, 1996

Food and Drug Administration: Roche Laboratories announces withdrawal of Posicor from the market (FDA Talk Paper T98-33). Rockville, MD, National Press Office, June 8, 1998 [www.fda.gov/opacom/hpwhats.html]

Food and Drug Administration: Janssen Pharmaceutica stops marketing cisapride in the US (FDA Talk Paper T00-14). Rockville, MD, National Press Office, March 23, 2000 [www.fda.gov/opacom/hpwhats.html]

Fuhr U: Drug interactions with grapefruit juice: extent, probable mechanism and clinical relevance. Drug Saf 18:251–272, 1998

Guengerich FP: Cytochrome P-450 3A4: regulation and the role in drug metabolism. Annu Rev Pharmacol Toxicol 39:1–17, 1999

Hukkinsen SK: Plasma concentrations of triazolam are increased by concomitant ingestion of grapefruit juice. Clin Pharmacol Ther 58:127–131, 1995

Ishizaki T, Horai Y: Cytochrome P450 and the metabolism of proton pump inhibitors—emphasis on rabeprazole (review article). Aliment Pharmacol Ther 13 (suppl 3):27–36, 1999

Johne A, Brockmoller J, Bauer S, et al: Pharmacokinetic interaction of digoxin with an herbal extract from St John's wort *(Hypericum perforatum)*. Clin Pharmacol Ther 66:338–345, 1999

Karliova M, Treichel U, Malago M, et al: Interaction of *Hypericum perforatum* (St. John's wort) with cyclosporin A metabolism in a patient after liver transplantation. 33:853–855, 2000

Keogh A, Spratt P, McCosker C, et al: Ketoconazole to reduce the need for cyclosporine after cardiac transplantation. N Engl J Med 333:628–633, 1995

Ketter TA, Flockhart DA, Post RM, et al: The emerging role of cytochrome P450 3A in psychopharmacology. J Clin Psychopharmacol 15:387–398, 1995

Ketter TA, Frye MA, Cora-Locatelli G, et al: Metabolism and excretion of mood stabilizers and new anticonvulsants. Cell Mol Neurobiol 19:511–532, 1999

Kivisto KT, Lamberg TS, Kantola T, et al: Plasma buspirone concentrations are greatly increased by erythromycin and itraconazole. Clin Pharmacol Ther 62:348–354, 1997

Kosuge K, Nishimoto M, Kimura M, et al: Enhanced effect of triazolam with diltiazem. Br J Clin Pharmacol 43:367–372, 1997

Levy RH: Cytochrome P450 isoenzymes and antiepileptic drugs. Epilepsia 36 (suppl 5):S8–S13, 1995

Lu ML, Lane HY, Chen KP, et al: Fluvoxamine reduces the clozapine dosage needed in refractory schizophrenic patients. J Clin Psychiatry 61:594–599, 2000

Monsarrat B, Chatelut E, Alvinerie P, et al: Modification of paclitaxel metabolism by drug induction of cytochrome P450A4 in a cancer patient (abstract). Proceedings of the Annual Meeting of the American Association for Cancer Research 38:A31, 1997

Moore LB, Goodwin B, Jones SA, et al: St. John's wort induces hepatic drug metabolism through activation of the pregnane X receptor. Proc Natl Acad Sci U S A 97:7500–7502, 2000

Moore LW, Alloway RR, Acchiardo SR, et al: Clinical observations of metabolic changes occurring in renal transplant recipients receiving ketoconazole. Transplantation 61:537–541, 1996

Norvir package insert. Chicago, IL, Abbott Laboratories, 1996

Ouellet D, Hsu A, Qian J, et al: Effect of ritonavir on the pharmacokinetics of ethinyl oestradiol in healthy female volunteers. Br J Clin Pharmacol 46:111–116, 1998

Owen JR, Nemeroff CB: New antidepressants and the cytochrome P450 system: focus on venlafaxine, nefazodone, and mirtazapine. Depress Anxiety 7 (suppl 1):24–32, 1998

Pichard L, Fabre I, Daujat M, et al: Effect of corticosteroids on the expression of cytochromes P450 and on cyclosporin A oxidase activity in primary cultures of human hepatocytes. Mol Pharmacol 41:1047–1055, 1992

Piscitelli SC, Kress DR, Bertz RJ, et al: The effect of ritonavir on the pharmacokinetics of meperidine and normeperidine. Pharmacotherapy 20:549–553, 2000

Propulsid (drug warning). Titusville, NJ, Janssen Pharmaceutica, January 2000

Provigil package insert. West Chester, PA, Cephalon, Inc., 1999

Roby CA, Anderson GD, Kantor E, et al: St. John's wort: effect on CYP3A4 activity. Clin Pharmacol Ther 67:451–457, 2000

Ruschitzka F, Meier PJ, Turina M, et al: Acute heart transplant rejection due to Saint John's wort (letter). Lancet 355:548–549, 2000

Serzone package insert. Princeton, NJ, Bristol-Myers Squibb, 1995

Strayhorn VA, Baciewicz AM, Self TH: Update on rifampin drug interactions, III. Arch Intern Med 157:2453–2458, 1997

Szymanski S, Lieberman JA, Picou D, et al: A case-report of cimetidine induced clozapine toxicity. J Clin Psychiatry 52:21–22, 1991

Tanaka E: Gender-related differences in pharmacokinetics and their clinical significance. J Clin Pharm Ther 24:339–346, 1999

Tokinaga N, Kondo T, Kaneko S, et al: Hallucinations after a therapeutic dose of benzodiazepine hypnotics with co-administration of erythromycin. Psychiatry Clin Neurosci 50:337–339, 1996

Tseng AL, Foisy MM: Management of drug interactions in patients with HIV. Ann Pharmacother 31:1040–1058, 1997 von Moltke LL, Greenblatt DJ, Grassi JM, et al: Protease inhibitors as inhibitors of human cytochrome P450: high risk associated with ritonavir. J Clin Pharmacol 38:106–111, 1998

Von Rosensteil NA, Adam D: Macrolide antibiotic drug interactions of clinical significance. Drug Saf 13:105–122, 1995

Weber A, Jager R, Borner A, et al: Can grapefruit juice influence ethinyl-estradiol bioavailability? Contraception 53:41–47, 1996

Westlind A, Lofberg L, Tindberg N, et al: Interindividual differences in hepatic expression of CYP3A4: relationship to genetic polymorphism in the 5′-upstream regulatory region. Biochem Biophys Res Commun 259:201–205, 1999

Wetzel H, Anghelescu I, Szegedi A, et al: Pharmacokinetic interactions of clozapine with selective serotonin reuptake inhibitors: differential effects of fluvoxamine and paroxetine in a prospective study. J Clin Psychopharmacol 18:2–9, 1998

Zhang QY, Dunbar D, Ostrooska A, et al: Characterization of human small intestinal cytochromes P-450. Drug Metab Dispos 27:804–809, 1999

■ STUDY CASES

Vignette 1

A 37-year-old Caucasian man who had tested positive for the human immunodeficiency virus (HIV) was severely depressed and began nortriptyline therapy. He improved clinically at a dose of 75 mg/day, and the serum tricyclic level was 87 ng/mL (therapeutic range, 50–150 ng/mL). His infectious disease physician prescribed ritonavir and saquinavir. The psychiatrist was notified about the new medication and told the patient to obtain a tricyclic level measurement 5–7 days after initiation of treatment with ritonavir and saquinavir. The patient did so and returned complaining of increasing depressive symptoms. His serum tricyclic level was 203 ng/mL.

Comment

3A4 and 2D6 inhibition: The psychiatrist and infectious disease physician correctly anticipated that ritonavir and saquinavir might increase tricyclic levels. Indeed, the tricyclic level increased beyond the therapeutic range, which may have reduced nortriptyline's effectiveness. The presumed mechanism for this interaction is ritonavir's potent inhibition of several P450 enzymes, including 2D6, 3A4, 2C9, and 2C19. Nortriptyline is metabolized by 2D6, 3A4, and perhaps other enzymes. Additionally, saquinavir modestly inhibits 3A4.

The patient moved away from the area, and nortriptyline levels after 4 weeks of therapy were not obtained. If ritonavir induced nortriptyline metabolism, this would have occurred after several weeks, requiring another dose adjustment.

References

Tseng AL, Foisy MM: Management of drug interactions in patients with HIV. Ann Pharmacother 31:1040–1058, 1997

Venkatakrishnan K, von Moltke LL, Greenblatt DJ: Nortriptyline E-10-hydroxylation in vitro is mediated by human CYP2D6 (high affinity) and CYP3A4 (low affinity): implications for interactions with enzyme-inducing drugs. J Clin Pharmacol 39:567–577, 1999

Vignette 2

A 38-year-old HIV-positive Caucasian man with several chronic problems, including allergic rhinitis, degenerative joint disease, and gastroesophageal reflux, began nelfinavir and nevirapine therapy. He became increasingly depressed, and treatment with doxepin was begun. Over time, the doxepin dose was titrated to 300 mg/day, with few side effects and questionable efficacy, despite good compliance. Serum tricyclic levels were low, ranging from 35 to 50 ng/mL. Viral load suppression was never achieved, and the patient's CD4 count continued to decrease.

Comment

3A4 induction: Nelfinavir has only mild inhibitory effects on 3A4 and 1A2. However, nevirapine induces 3A4. Although the metabolism of doxepin has not been studied as well as the metabolisms of other tertiary tricyclics (amitriptyline and imipramine), the drug is probably metabolized similarly—primarily by 3A4 and secondarily by other enzymes. Nevirapine likely induced the metabolism of doxepin, causing low tricyclic levels despite a relatively high dose of doxepin. Nelfinavir is also metabolized at 3A4, and nevirapine was probably inducing the protease inhibitor, placing this patient at risk for viral resistance to all protease inhibitors.

References

Lemoine A, Gautier JC, Azoulay D, et al: Major pathway of imipramine metabolism is catalyzed by cytochromes P-450 1A2 and P-450 3A4 in human liver. Mol Pharmacol 43:827–832, 1993

Tseng AL, Foisy MM: Management of drug interactions in patients with HIV. Ann Pharmacother 31:1040–1058, 1997

Venkatakrishnan K, Greenblatt DJ, von Moltke LL, et al: Five distinct human cytochromes mediate amitriptyline *N*-demethylation in vitro: dominance of CYP 2C19 and 3A4. J Clin Pharmacol 38:112–121, 1998

Vignette 3

A 35-year-old HIV-positive African American man had been taking fluoxetine (20 mg/day) for several years and ritonavir for several months without problems. The patient tried his mother's zolpidem (10 mg) because of sleeplessness. He slept for 14 hours and had a "hangover" the next day.

Comment

3A4 inhibition: Zolpidem is metabolized by 3A4. Ritonavir potently inhibits 3A4, and fluoxetine also inhibits 3A4, though not as potently. It is likely that this inhibition caused a delay in zolpidem's clearance, leading to the enhanced effect.

References

Tseng AL, Foisy MM: Management of drug interactions in patients with HIV. Ann Pharmacother 31:1040–1058, 1997

von Moltke LL, Greenblatt DJ, Granda BW, et al: Zolpidem metabolism in vitro: responsible cytochromes, chemical inhibitors, and in vivo correlations. Br J Clin Pharmacol 48:89–97, 1999

Vignette 4

A 45-year-old Caucasian man with chronic schizophrenia was being treated with haloperidol decanoate at a stable dose of 200 mg/month. He developed a seizure disorder and was prescribed phenytoin by his neurologist. Within 2 months, the patient's psychotic symptoms worsened, and he required hospitalization. Although baseline haloperidol levels had not been obtained before initiation of phenytoin therapy, a haloperidol level obtained in the hospital while the patient was receiving both haloperidol and phenytoin was low (less than 2 ng/mL).

Comment

3A4 inhibition: Haloperidol is metabolized by several P450 enzymes, including 3A4, and by phase II enzymes. Phenytoin induces 3A4. It is likely that over several weeks, phenytoin induced 3A4 and decreased serum haloperidol levels, leading to a recurrence of psychotic symptoms.

References

Kudo S, Ishizaki T: Pharmacokinetics of haloperidol: an update. Clin Pharmacokinet 37:435–456, 1999

Linnoila M, Viukari M, Vaisanen K: Effect of anticonvulsants on plasma haloperidol and thioridazine levels. Am J Psychiatry 137:819–821,1980

■ DRUGS METABOLIZED BY 3A4

Antidepressants

Amitriptyline[1]
Citalopram[2]
Clomipramine[1]
Fluoxetine
Mirtazapine[2]
Nefazodone
Paroxetine[2]
Reboxetine
Sertraline[2]
Trazodone[2,3]
Venlafaxine[2]

Antipsychotics

Clozapine[4]
Haloperidol[5]
Pimozide[6]
Quetiapine[7]

Sedative-hypnotics

Benzodiazepines

Diazepam[2]
Nitrazepam[2]

Triazolobenzodiazepines

Alprazolam
Estazolam
Midazolam
Triazolam

Other sedative-hypnotics

Zaleplon
Zolpidem

Other drugs

Analgesics

Alfentanil[2]
Codeine[2]
Fentanyl
Methadone[2]
Sufentanil
Tramadol[2]

Antiarrhythmics[6]

Amiodarone
Lidocaine
Propafenone[2]
Quinidine

Antibiotics (miscellaneous)

Ciprofloxacin
Rifabutin
Rifampin
Sparfloxacin[2]

Antiepileptics

Carbamazepine
Tiagabine[2]
Valproic acid[2]

DRUGS METABOLIZED BY 3A4 (continued)

Other drugs

Antimalarials
Chloroquine
Halofantrine[6]
Primaquine

Antineoplastics
Bulsulfan
Cyclophosphamide[2]
Daunorubicin
Docetaxel
Doxorubicin
Etoposide
Ifosfamide[2]
Paclitaxel[2]
Tamoxifen[2]
Teniposide
Toremifene[2]
Trofosfamide
Vinblastine
Vincristine
Vindesine
Vinorelbine

Other drugs

Antiparkinsonian drugs
Bromocriptine
Pergolide
Ropinirole[2]

Antirejection drugs
Cyclosporine
Rapamycin
Tacrolimus

Calcium-channel blockers
Amlodipine
Diltiazem[2]
Felodipine
Nicardipine
Nifedipine
Nimodipine[2]
Nitrendipine
Verapamil[2]

Other drugs

HMG-CoA reductase inhibitors
Atorvastatin
Cerivastatin
Lovastatin
Simvastatin

Macrolide antibiotics
Azithromycin
Clarithromycin
Dirithromycin
Erythromycin
Rokitamycin
Troleandomycin

Nonnucleoside reverse transcriptase inhibitors
Delavirdine[2]
Efavirenz
Nevirapine[2]

Nonsedating antihistamines
Astemizole[6,8]
Ebastine[6]
Loratadine[7]
Terfenadine[6,8]

■ DRUGS METABOLIZED BY 3A4 (continued)

Other drugs	Other drugs	Other drugs
Protease inhibitors (antivirals)	*Miscellaneous drugs*	*Steroids*
Amprenavir	Acetaminophen[2]	Cortisol
Indinavir	Carvedilol[2]	Dexamethasone
Lopinavir	Cilostazol[2]	Ethinyl estradiol
Nelfinavir	Cisapride	Prednisone
Ritonavir	Cyclobenzaprine[10]	Progesterone
Saquinavir	Ergots	Testosterone
Proton pump inhibitors	Ketoconazole	
Lansoprazole[9]	Metoprolol[2]	
Omeprazole[9]	Montelukast	
Pantoprazole[9]	Ondansetron[2]	
Rabeprazole	Sildenafil	
Psychotropic drugs, other	Sibutramine	
Buspirone	Vesnarinone	
Donepezil[2]		

■ DRUGS METABOLIZED BY 3A4 *(continued)*

Note. HMG-CoA = hydroxymethylglutaryl–coenzyme A.

[1]Tertiary tricyclics are metabolized preferentially by 3A4 but are also metabolized by 2D6, 1A2, 2C9, and 2C19.

[2]Also significantly metabolized by other P450 enzymes.

[3]Metabolized by 3A4 to *m*-chlorophenylpiperazine.

[4]Also metabolized by 1A2 and, to a lesser extent, 2D6.

[5]Also metabolized by 2D6 and 1A2.

[6]Potentially toxic to the cardiac conduction system at high levels and therefore should not be used with potent inhibitors of 3A4.

[7]Also metabolized by 2D6.

[8]No longer available in the United States.

[9]Also metabolized by 2C19.

[10]Also metabolized by 1A2.

■ INHIBITORS OF 3A4

Antidepressants	Antimicrobials	Other inhibitors
Selective serotonin reuptake inhibitors[1]	*Antibiotics, other*	Anastrozole
Citalopram[c]	Ciprofloxacin[3,a]	Bromocriptine
Fluoxetine	Norfloxacin[4]	Chloroquine
Fluvoxamine	Quinupristin/dalfopristin[2,a]	Cimetidine[8]
Norfluoxetine	Sparfloxacin[4]	Cisapride
Paroxetine	*Azole antifungals*	Cyclosporine[b]
Sertraline	Fluconazole[5]	Diltiazem
Other antidepressants	Itraconazole[2,a]	Grapefruit juice[2,4,a]
Nefazodone[2,a]	Ketoconazole[2,6,a]	Methadone[a,b]
	Miconazole	Methylprednisone
	Macrolide antibiotics	Mibefradil[2,9,a]
	Clarithromycin[2,a]	Nifedipine
	Erythromycin[2,a]	Primaquine
	(Others less inhibitory)	Tamoxifen
	Nonnucleoside reverse transcriptase inhibitors	Valproic acid
	Delavirdine[a,b]	Verapamil
	Efavirenz[2,a]	Zafirlukast[10]

■ INHIBITORS OF 3A4 (continued)

Antimicrobials
Protease inhibitors
Indinavir[2,a]
Lopinavir/ritonavir[11]
Ritonavir[2,7,a]
(Others less inhibitory)

[1] Also inhibit other P450 enzymes.
[2] Has demonstrated strong inhibition and should be used with caution with other drugs metabolized by 3A4.
[3] Also a potent inhibitor of 1A2.
[4] Also an inhibitor of 1A2.
[5] Potent inhibitor of 2C9.
[6] Also an inhibitor of 2C19.
[7] Also a potent inhibitor of 2D6, 2C9, and 2C19.
[8] Also an inhibitor of 2D6, 1A2, and 2C9.
[9] Also a potent inhibitor of 2D6; no longer available in the United States.
[10] Also an inhibitor of 1A2 and 2C9.
[11] Trade name Kaletra.

[a] Potent (bold type).
[b] Moderate.
[c] Mild.

■ INDUCERS OF 3A4

Antiepileptics	Other inducers
Carbamazepine[2,a]	Cisplatin
Oxcarbazepine	Cyclophosphamide
Phenobarbital[2,a]	Dexamethasone
Phenytoin[2,a]	Efavirenz
Primidone	Ifosfamide
	?**Lopinavir/ritonavir**[1,4]
	Methylprednisolone
	Modafinil
	Nevirapine
	Prednisone
	Rifampin[2,a]
	Rifapentine[2,a]
	Ritonavir[4]
	St. John's wort
	Troglitazone[3]

[1]Trade name Kaletra.
[2]Are "pan-inducers"—also induce most other P450 enzymes.
[3]Removed from U.S. market.
[4]Ritonavir currently know to induce only 3A4.

[a]Potent (bold type).
[b]Moderate.
[c]Mild.

6

1A2

P450 1A2 is recognized as an important enzyme in human metabolism (Brosen 1995). It has long been identified as the primary enzyme involved in the metabolism of methylxanthines, such as caffeine and theophylline.

■ WHAT DOES 1A2 DO?

1A2 is involved in phase I metabolism of substances. Its actions are primarily hydroxylation and demethylation of compounds. 1A2 also metabolizes some endogenous compounds, such as estradiol-17β and uroporphyrinogen. Men appear to have slightly more activity than do women.

■ WHERE IS 1A2?

1A2 is found exclusively in the liver. The enzyme accounts for 10%–15% of enzyme activity in the liver.

■ DOES 1A2 HAVE ANY POLYMORPHISMS?

Whether 1A2 has any polymorphisms has not been clearly elucidated. There does seem to be a 40-fold difference in enzyme activity in humans (Guengerich et al. 1999), but it is not clear whether this difference is due to environmental factors of inhibition and induction. There have been some reports of genetic polymorphisms in Asians (rare poor metabolizers) and possible genetic polymorphisms in

Caucasians (extensive metabolizers), but clinical significance is currently uncertain. We expect that more information will be obtained on the polymorphic character of this enzyme in the next few years. The *1A2* gene is located on chromosome 15.

■ ARE THERE DRUGS THAT INHIBIT 1A2 ACTIVITY?

Yes. Fluvoxamine and ciprofloxacin are the two most common medications in use that inhibit 1A2. Other fluoroquinolone antibiotics (Caspi 1998; Markowitz et al. 1997; Mizuki et al. 1996) and grapefruit juice (Fuhr 1998) are also inhibitory (the latter by a different mechanism than its effect on 3A4), and such inhibition may have clinical significance if the aforementioned are given with drugs with relatively narrow therapeutic windows. Fortunately, not many drugs appear to be primarily or exclusively metabolized by this enzyme. The only drugs that strongly depend on 1A2 are the methylxanthines, such as caffeine and theophylline (Miners and Birkett 1996). For this reason, caffeine and theophylline have been used as probes for 1A2 activity. Theophylline's dependence on 1A2 for metabolism is responsible for reports of a 70% decrease in clearance (Rasmussen et al. 1997) and resulting toxicity when the drug is administered with fluvoxamine (DeVane et al. 1997) or ciprofloxacin (Batty et al. 1995). We think that caffeine toxicity associated with administration of inhibitors of 1A2 is probably underreported because clinicians and patients alike do not recognize that patients' jitters are caused by increased levels of caffeine and are not a side effect of the therapeutic drug.

Other drugs that inhibit 1A2 are the antiarrhythmics mexiletine (Nakajima et al. 1998) and propafenone (Kobayashi et al 1998; Spinler et al. 1993), as well as the leukotriene antagonist zafirlukast (Katial et al. 1998). Propafenone and zafirlukast have been shown to increase theophylline levels.

Fluvoxamine is the most potent psychotropic inhibitor of this enzyme. Haloperidol, clozapine, imipramine, and theophylline levels have all been reported to increase three to six times above baseline (Brosen 1995). When given with clozapine, fluvoxamine must be used very cautiously, because it inhibits 3A4 and 1A2 potently and 2D6 moderately. All three of these enzymes are responsible for clozapine metabolism. (See Chapter 5 for more discussion.)

One study of fluvoxamine 100 mg/day for 6 days followed by a single 40-mg dose of tacrine revealed a decrease in oral clearance of tacrine of 730% (Becquemont et al. 1997). Caution is of course advised, because tacrine's main route of elimination is through 1A2. In addition, theophylline toxicity has been reported with concomitant use of fluvoxamine (Rasmussen et al. 1997), and the half-life of caffeine was increased from 5 to 31 hours with fluvoxamine administration (Jeppesen et al. 1996).

■ ARE THERE DRUGS THAT INDUCE 1A2 ACTIVITY?

Yes. Clinically, this is the most important fact to remember about this enzyme.

The most important inducer of 1A2 with clinical significance is tobacco smoke (Schrenk et al. 1998; Zevin and Benowitz 1999). Any drug metabolized by 1A2 will be used at higher doses in smokers, because the enzyme is already induced. We suspect that this fact is usually not recognized by the clinician. When a patient stops smoking (an action that is often encouraged), drug toxicity may occur. Because it takes a few weeks for induction (and, conversely, the dissipation of induction) to occur, cessation of smoking may result in increased drug levels several weeks later. Drugs such as theophylline, clozapine, and olanzapine are partially metabolized (30% or more) by 1A2 (Lyon 1999), and toxic levels may be reached when smoking is stopped. After cessation of smoking, several patients being treated with long-term clozapine therapy by one of the authors (S.C.A.) required decreases of clozapine doses to avoid toxicity. Monitoring serum levels during these transition periods is recommended.

Olanzapine is metabolized by several pathways, including 1A2 (30%–40%), glucuronidation by phase II enzymes, and, to a minor degree, 2D6 (Calleghan et al. 1999). Studies have indicated that smokers may need higher doses to achieve desired effects, because smoking increases clearance of olanzapine by as much as 40%. On a more theoretical level, we wonder whether it is wise for psychiatric facilities to require smoking cessation in the case of long inpatient stays. Patients typically resume smoking when discharged—which may lead to lowered serum levels of newly prescribed drugs.

Some inducers of 1A2 are not medications. Brussels sprouts, broccoli, cabbage, and other cruciferous vegetables, if eaten daily, will induce this enzyme (Jefferson 1998; Jefferson and Griest 1996; Kall et al. 1996), and cooking does not negate this effect. In addition, daily consumption of charbroiled foods (burned meats) will result in induction of this enzyme. The average American diet will typically not lead to induction of 1A2.

■ REFERENCES

Batty KT, Davis TM, Ilett KF, et al: The effect of ciprofloxacin on theophylline pharmacokinetics in healthy subjects. Br J Clin Pharmacol 39:305–311, 1995

Becquemont L, Ragueneau I, Le Bot MA, et al: Influence of the CYP1A2 inhibitor fluvoxamine on tacrine pharmacokinetics in humans. Clin Pharmacol Ther 61:619–627, 1997

Bloomer JC, Clarke SE, Chenery RJ: In vitro identification of the P450 enzymes responsible for the metabolism of ropinirole. Drug Metab Dispos 25:1–11, 1997

Brosen K: Drug interactions and the cytochrome P450 system: the role of cytochrome P450 1A2. Clin Pharmacokinet 29 (suppl 1):20–25, 1995

Calleghan JT, Bergstrom RF, Ptak LR, et al: Olanzapine: pharmacokinetic and pharmacodynamic profile. Clin Pharmacokinet 37:177–193, 1999

Caspi A: Therapeutic advantages of the newer fluoroquinolones. Pharmacy and Therapeutics 23:18–28, 1998

DeVane CL, Markowitz JS, Hardesty SJ, et al: Fluvoxamine-induced theophylline toxicity. Am J Psychiatry 154:1317–1318, 1997

Fuhr U: Drug interactions with grapefruit juice: extent, probable mechanism and clinical relevance. Drug Saf 18:251–272, 1998

Guengerich FP, Parileh A, Turesky RJ, et al: Inter-individual differences in the metabolism of environmental toxicants: cytochrome P450 1A2 as a prototype. Mutat Res 428:115–124, 1999

Jefferson JW: Drug and diet interactions: avoiding therapeutic paralysis. J Clin Psychiatry 59 (suppl 16):31–39, 1998

Jefferson JW, Griest JH: Brussels sprouts and psychopharmacology: understanding the cytochrome P450 enzyme system. Psychiatry Clin North Am: Annual on Drug Therapy 3:205–222, 1996

Jeppesen U, Loft S, Poulson HE, et al: A fluvoxamine-caffeine interaction study. Pharmacogenetics 6:213–222, 1996

Kall MA, Vang O, Clausen J: Effects of dietary broccoli on human in vivo drug metabolizing enzymes: evaluation of caffeine, oestrone and chlorzoxazone metabolism. Carcinogenesis 17:793–799, 1996

Katial RK, Stelzle RC, Bonner MW, et al: A drug interaction between zafirlukast and theophylline. Arch Intern Med 158:1713–1715, 1998

Kobayashi K, Nakajima M, Chiba K, et al: Inhibitory effects of antiarrhythmic drugs on phenacetin O-demethylation catalysed by human CYP1A2. Br J Clin Pharmacol 45:361–368, 1998

Lyon ER: A review of the effects of nicotine on schizophrenia and antipsychotic medications. Psychiatr Serv 50:1346–1350, 1999

Markowitz JS, Gill HS, DeVane CL, et al: Fluoroquinolone inhibition of clozapine metabolism (letter). Am J Psychiatry 154:881, 1997

Miners JO, Birkett DJ: The use of caffeine as a metabolic probe for human drug metabolizing enzymes. Gen Pharmacol 27:245–249, 1996

Mizuki Y, Fujiwara I, Yamaguchi T: Pharmacokinetic interactions related to the chemical structures of fluoroquinolones. J Antimicrob Chemother 37 (suppl A):41–55, 1996

Nakajima M, Kobayashi K, Shimada N, et al: Involvement of CYP1A2 in mexiletine metabolism. Br J Clin Pharmacol 46:55–62, 1998

Rasmussen BB, Jeppesen U, Gaist D, et al: Griseofulvin and fluvoxamine interactions with the metabolism of theophylline. Ther Drug Monit 19:56–62, 1997

Schrenk D, Brockmeier D, Morike K, et al: A distribution of CYP1A2 phenotypes among smokers and non-smokers in a cohort of healthy volunteers. Eur J Clin Pharmacol 53:361–367, 1998

Spinler SA, Gammaitoni A, Charland SL, et al: Propafenone-theophylline interaction. Pharmacotherapy 13:68–71, 1993

Zevin S, Benowitz NL: Drug interactions with tobacco smoking: an update. Clin Pharmacokinet 36:425–438, 1999

■ STUDY CASES

Vignette 1

A 35-year-old Caucasian woman with major depression and/or bipolar disorder and multiple psychiatric hospitalizations failed to respond to numerous treatments, including electroconvulsive therapy. Her fluvoxamine dose was titrated to 300 mg/day, without much benefit. Psychotic symptoms began to predominate. Her clozapine dose was titrated to 200 mg/day over several weeks. The patient began to complain of dizziness and had mild hypotension. Her serum clozapine level was 1,950 ng/mL, and a confirmatory measurement revealed a level of 2,040 ng/mL. Fluvoxamine therapy was discontinued, and clozapine levels were closely monitored. Three days after discontinuation of fluvoxamine therapy, the clozapine level had decreased to 693 ng/mL, and on the fifth day after cessation of treatment with fluvoxamine, the level was 175 ng/mL. The aforementioned side effects disappeared.

Comment

1A2 inhibition: Fluvoxamine potently inhibits several P450 enzymes, including 1A2, 2C9, and 2C19. It also moderately inhibits 3A4. Clozapine is metabolized by 1A2 and, to some extent, 3A4 and 2D6. This case and others reported in the literature indicate just how much fluvoxamine can increase clozapine levels. The case also illustrates how quickly inhibition can be reversed when treatment with the offending inhibitor (here, fluvoxamine) is discontinued.

References

Armstrong SC, Stephans JR: Blood clozapine levels elevated by fluvoxamine: potential for side effects and lower clozapine dosage. J Clin Psychiatry 58:499, 1997

Wetzel H, Anghelescu I, Szegedi A, et al: Pharmacokinetic interactions of clozapine and selective serotonin reuptake inhibitors: differential effects of fluvoxamine and paroxetine in a prospective study. J Clin Psychopharmacol 18:2–9, 1998

Vignette 2

A 48-year-old Caucasian man with schizophrenia was effectively treated with clozapine 500 mg/day. The patient was a longtime smoker but was able to spontaneously stop smoking 2 years after the clozapine dose was established. Several weeks after smoking cessation, the patient complained of some side effects that were attributed to the clozapine, including sedation and constipation. Serum clozapine levels were found to be more than 700 ng/mL, nearly twice what the clozapine levels had been when the patient was smoking.

Comment

1A2 induction: The major P450 enzyme involved in metabolism of clozapine is 1A2, although 3A4 and 2D6 are also involved. Smoking induces 1A2. When smoking ceases, 1A2 activity returns to normal after 3–6 weeks. Patients taking drugs such as clozapine have increased serum levels several weeks after cessation of smoking.

Reference

Seppala NH, Leinonen EV, Lehtonen ML, et al: Clozapine serum concentrations are lower in smoking than non-smoking schizophrenic patients. Pharmacol Toxicol 85:244–246, 1999

■ DRUGS METABOLIZED BY 1A2

Antidepressants	Antipsychotics	Other drugs	
Amitriptyline[1]	Clozapine[3]	Caffeine	Phenacetin
Clomipramine[1]	Haloperidol[2]	Cyclobenzaprine[5]	Propranolol[2]
Fluvoxamine[2]	Olanzapine[4]	Dacarbazine[2]	Ropinorole[6]
Imipramine[1]		Flutamide	Tacrine
Mirtazapine[2]		Grepafloxacin	Theophylline
		Mexiletine[2]	Toremifene[2]
		Ondansetron[2]	Verapamil[7]
		Pentoxifylline	R-Warfarin[8]

[1]Tertiary tricyclic antidepressants are demethylated by 1A2 and metabolized by 3A4, 2C9, 2C19, and 2D6.
[2]Metabolized by other P450 enzymes as well.
[3]Also metabolized by 3A4 and 2D6.
[4]Metabolized (30%–40%) by 1A2, as well as by phase II (50% through glucuronidation) and 2D6.
[5]Also metabolized by 3A4.
[6]Also metabolized secondarily by 3A4.
[7]Metabolized primarily by 3A4.
[8]The weaker pharmacological isomer of warfarin (see Chapter 7).

■ INHIBITORS OF 1A2

Fluoroquinolone antibiotics	Selective serotonin reuptake inhibitors	Other inhibitors
Ciprofloxacin[a]	**Fluvoxamine**[a]	Anastrozole
Enoxacin[a]		Cimetidine
Grepafloxacin		Flutamide[1]
Norfloxacin		Grapefruit juice[2,b]
Ofloxacin		Lidocaine
Sparfloxacin		**Mexiletine**[a]
		Propafenone[a]
		Ranitidine
		Rifampin
		Ropinirole
		Tacrine
		Tocainide
		Zafirlukast[b]

[1]Flutamide's primary metabolite is a potent inhibitor of 1A2.
[2]Inhibits primarily 3A4 in the gut wall. 1A2 inhibition is milder and its mechanism is unknown.

[a]Potent (bold type).
[b]Moderate.
[c]Mild.

■ INDUCERS OF 1A2

Drugs	Foods	Other inducers
Caffeine	Broccoli	Chronic smoking
Carbamazepine	Brussels sprouts	
Griseofulvin	Cabbage	
Lansoprazole[c]	Cauliflower	
Moricizine	Charbroiled or burned foods	
Omeprazole		
Rifampin		

[a]Potent (bold type).
[b]Moderate.
[c]Mild.

7

2C9

2C9 is under increasing scrutiny because recent evidence indicates that the enzyme is polymorphic. The list of drugs metabolized by 2C9 is not large, but it is growing (Miners and Birkett 1998). Often the enzyme is listed as 2C8, 2C9, or 2C10 in older literature. These three enzymes are very similar, and in general it is not clinically useful to distinguish between them.

■ WHAT DOES 2C9 DO?

2C9's actions, like those of other P450 enzymes, include hydroxylation, demethylation, and dealkylation of compounds. Also like other P450 enzymes, 2C9 metabolizes substrates that are endogenous compounds. 2C9 alone metabolizes liver arachidonic acid (Rifkind et al. 1995).

■ WHERE IS 2C9?

2C9 is found in many tissues, but it plays its role in drug metabolism in the liver. Along with its cousin 2C19, it accounts for about 20% of P450 activity in the liver.

■ DOES 2C9 HAVE ANY POLYMORPHISMS?

Yes. 2C8, 2C9, and 2C10 are all located in the same subchromosomal region on chromosome 10 (Inoue et al. 1994). Recent studies indicate that 2C9 has a poor metabolizer (PM) polymorphism. Drugs dependent on 2C9 for metabolism (such as warfarin, tolbutamide, and phenytoin) (Chiba 1998; Coutts and Urichuk 1999) may have decreased metabolism in PMs. Hence, as with 2D6 and 2C19, the terms *extensive* or rapid (average) *metabolizer* and *poor metabolizer* are beginning to be used to refer clinically to the two variants. Two percent of Japanese and 6%–9% of Caucasians are PMs at 2C9. Although there are currently no recognized substrate probes for determining clinical phenotypic variability of 2C9, several drugs are strong possibilities, including tolbutamide (Miners and Birkett 1996), phenytoin (Aynacioglu et al. 1999), and naproxen (Moody et al. 1999). The full clinical significance of this polymorphism is unclear.

■ ARE THERE DRUGS THAT INHIBIT 2C9 ACTIVITY?

Yes. Of the selective serotonin inhibitors (SSRIs), fluvoxamine is the most potent inhibitor; other SSRIs minimally inhibit 2C9 (Hemeryck et al. 1999). Nonpsychotropic drugs, including zafirlukast, some sulfonamides, ritonavir, and fluconazole, make up the remainder of the list of inhibitors. The latter two drugs are inhibitors of 3A4 as well.

2C9 inhibition has not received the same attention in the literature as 2D6 and 3A4. The paucity of information is due to the small number of drugs exclusively metabolized by 2C9. Also, drugs partially or fully metabolized by 2C9 do not, in general, have dire consequences if their metabolism is impeded by an inhibitor.

Substrates with adverse outcomes if inhibited at 2C9 or if administered to a PM at 2C9 are warfarin, phenytoin, and the nonsteroidal anti-inflammatory drugs (NSAIDs).

Warfarin

S-Warfarin is the more active isomer of the racemic mix of warfarin. *S*-Warfarin is metabolized primarily by 2C9 (*R*-warfarin is metabolized by 1A2). Studies have indicated that this interaction may be behind fluvoxamine's role in increasing clotting times in patients treated with warfarin. Although other SSRIs have been reported to have a similar effect on clotting times, the mechanism may not be inhibition of 2C9 (data on file, Solvay Pharmaceuticals, Inc., Marietta, GA; Hemeryck et al. 1999).

Phenytoin

By 1994, there were 23 reported cases of significantly increased phenytoin levels when the drug was concomitantly administered with fluoxetine (Nightingale 1994). Theoretically, fluvoxamine should inhibit phenytoin's metabolism; however, no case reports of such an interaction have yet been published. Additionally, fluconazole, an inhibitor of 3A4, also inhibits 2C9 (Black et al. 1996), and cases of increased phenytoin levels during fluconazole therapy have been reported (Cadle et al. 1994).

Nonsteroidal Anti-inflammatory Inhibitors

Although multiple studies have indicated that nearly all NSAIDs (including the newer cyclooxygenase-2 [Cox-2] inhibitors) depend on 2C9 for their metabolism, we did not find reports of adverse outcomes in PMs at 2C9 or in patients receiving 2C9 inhibitors concomitantly. This lack of reports may be due to the fact that NSAIDs have both wide therapeutic windows and alternative metabolic pathways (mainly phase II conjugation with glucuronic acid).

■ ARE THERE DRUGS THAT INDUCE 2C9 ACTIVITY?

Yes. The only clearly recognized inducer is rifampin. This drug was recognized as an inducer in the 1970s, although it was not until the mid-1990s that the actual enzyme induced was found to be 2C9 (its cousin 2C19 is also induced by rifampin). Rifampin has been shown to reduce serum levels, by induction, of warfarin (Heimark et al. 1987), tolbutamide (Zilly et al. 1977), and phenytoin (Kay et al. 1985)—all drugs very dependent on 2C9. Phenytoin and secobarbital may also induce 2C9.

82

■ REFERENCES

Aynacioglu AS, Brackmoller J, Bauer S, et al: Frequency of cytochrome P450 CYP2C9 variants in a Turkish population and the functional relevance for phenytoin. Br J Clin Pharmacol 48:409–415, 1999

Baldwin SJ, Bloomer JC, Smith GJ, et al: Ketoconazole and sulphaphenazole as the respective selective inhibitors of P4503A and 2C9. Xenobiotica 25:261–270, 1995

Black DJ, Kunze KL, Wienkers LC, et al: Warfarin-fluconazole, II: a metabolically based drug interaction—in vivo studies. Drug Metab Dispos 24:422–428, 1996

Cadle RM, Zenon GJ 3rd, Rodriguez-Barradas MC, et al: Fluconazole-induced symptomatic phenytoin toxicity. Ann Pharmacother 28:191–195, 1994

Chiba K: Genetic polymorphism of the CYP2C subfamily. Nippon Yakurigaku Zasshi 112:15–21, 1998

Coutts RT, Urichuk LJ: Polymorphic cytochromes P450 and drugs used in psychiatry. Cell Mol Neurobiol 19:325–354, 1999

Heimark LD, Gibaldi M, Trager WF, et al: The mechanism of the warfarin-rifampin drug interaction. Clin Pharmacol Ther 42:388–394, 1987

Hemeryck A, De Vriendt C, Belpaire FM: Inhibition of CYP2C9 by selective serotonin reuptake inhibitors: in vitro studies with tolbutamide and (S)-warfarin using human liver microsomes. Eur J Clin Pharmacol 54:947–951, 1999

Inoue K, Inazawa J, Suzuki Y, et al: Fluorescence in situ hybridization analysis of chromosomal localization of three human cytochrome P450 2C genes (CYP2C8, 2C9, 2C10) at 10q24.1. Jpn J Hum Genet 39:337–343, 1994

Kay L, Kampmann JP, Svendsen TL, et al: Influence of rifampicin and isoniazid on the kinetics of phenytoin. Br J Clin Pharmacol 20:323–326, 1985

Miners JO, Burkitt DJ: Use of tolbutamide as a substrate probe for human hepatic cytochrome P450 2C9. Methods Enzymol 272:139–145, 1996

Miners JO, Burkitt DJ: Cytochrome P4502C9: an enzyme of major importance in human drug metabolism. Br J Clin Pharmacol 45:525–538, 1998

Moody GC, Griffin SJ, Mather AN, et al: Fully automated analysis of activities catalysed by the major human liver cytochrome P450 (CYP) enzymes: assessment of human CYP inhibition potential. Xenobiotica 29:53–75, 1999

Nightingale SL: From the Food and Drug Administration. JAMA 271:1067, 1994

Rifkind AB, Lee C, Chang TK, et al: Arachidonic acid metabolism by human cytochrome P450s 2C8, 2C9, 2E1, and 1A2: regioselective oxygen-
ation and evidence for a role for CYP2C enzymes in arachidonic acid
epoxygenation in human liver microsomes. Arch Biochem Biophys
320:380–389, 1995

Zilly W, Breimer DD, Richter E: Stimulation of drug metabolism by rifampicin in patients with cirrhosis or cholestasis measured by increased
hexobarbital and tolbutamide clearance. Eur J Clin Pharmacol 11:287–
293, 1977

■ STUDY CASE

A 40-year-old Caucasian woman was prescribed fluoxetine 20 mg/
day for anxiety and depressive symptoms. She had been treated for
many years with phenytoin 300 mg/day for a seizure disorder, without significant side effects. After 1 week of fluoxetine therapy, she
complained of dizziness and somnolence. Serum phenytoin levels
were 30 μg/mL (reference range, 10–20 μg/mL).

Comment

2C9 and 2C19 inhibition: Phenytoin is metabolized by 2C9,
2C19, and phase II conjugation enzymes. Although not a potent inhibitor of 2C9 and 2C19, fluoxetine does inhibit these enzymes and
most certainly was the cause of this woman's increase in phenytoin
levels.

Reference

Nightingale SL: From the Food and Drug Administration. JAMA 271:1067,
1994

84

■ DRUGS METABOLIZED BY 2C9

Angiotensin II blockers	Hypoglycemics, oral	Nonsteroidal anti-inflammatory drugs	Other drugs
Losartan	Glipizide	Celecoxib[1]	Carmustine
Valsartan	Glyburide	Diclofenac	Paclitaxel[2]
	Rosiglitazone	Ibuprofen	Phenytoin
	Tolbutamide	Indomethacin	Tamoxifen
		Mefenamic acid	Tetrahydrocannabinol
		Naproxen	Torsemide
		Piroxicam	Tricyclic antidepressants[2]
		Suprofen	S-Warfarin[3]
			Zafirlukast

[1] A cyclooxygenase-2 (Cox-2) inhibitor.
[2] See Chapters 4 and 5.
[3] S-Warfarin is the more active isomer of warfarin. R-warfarin is metabolized by 1A2.

■ INHIBITORS OF 2C9

Selective serotonin reuptake inhibitors	Other inhibitors
Fluoxetine[b]	Amiodarone
Fluvoxamine[a]	Anastrozole
Paroxetine[c]	Cimetidine
Sertraline[c]	Clopidogrel
	Delavirdine
	Efavirenz
	Fluconazole[a]
	Isoniazid
	Modafinil
	Phenylbutazone
	Ranitidine
	Ritonavir[a]
	Sulfaphenazole[a]
	Sulfinpyrazone
	Zafirlukast

[a]Potent (bold type).
[b]Moderate.
[c]Mild.

■ INDUCERS OF 2C9

?Carbamazepine
Cyclophosphamide
Ifosfamide
?Phenobarbital
Phenytoin
Rifabutin
Rifampin
Rifapentine
Valproic acid

8

2C19

2C19 is a cousin of 2C9—only 43 of 490 amino acids differ (Jung et al. 1998). 2C19 is perhaps best known for its polymorphic distribution. Although 2C19 is related to 2C9, there are some significant differences between the two enzymes.

■ WHAT DOES 2C19 DO?

2C19 is involved in phase I metabolism of substances. Its actions, like those of other P450 enzymes, include hydroxylation, demethylation, and dealkylation of compounds.

■ WHERE IS 2C19?

2C19 is found in many tissues, but it plays its role in the metabolism of drugs in the liver. Together, 2C19 and 2C9 are responsible for approximately 20% of P450 activity in the liver.

■ DOES 2C19 HAVE ANY POLYMORPHISMS?

Yes. As with 2D6, there are two phenotypes: the poor metabolizer (PM) phenotype and the extensive (average) metabolizer phenotype. Racial differences abound with regard to 2C19 polymorphisms, and the number of population genetic studies is growing rapidly. In general, studies have revealed that 2%–6% of Caucasians, 15%–20% of Japanese, and 10%–20% of Africans are PMs (Flockhart 1995). But there is wide variability among populations.

For example, the percentage of Polynesians who are PMs ranges from 38% to 79%, depending on the location within Polynesia. This variability was discovered somewhat accidentally; patients from the Vanuatu Islands were reported to have high or toxic levels of proguanil, the antimalarial agent metabolized by 2C19 (side effects were nausea, vomiting, and diarrhea) (Kaneko et al. 1999).

S-Mephenytoin has long been used in the laboratory as a substrate probe for 2C19 activity (Wedlund et al. 1984; Wrighton et al. 1993). In fact, older literature often referred to 2C19 as the S-*mephenytoin enzyme.* Clinicians may want to measure the clearance of *S*-mephenytoin to establish 2C19 activity in their patients.

This phenotypic variability has clinical consequences, both good and bad. Aoyama et al. (1999) discovered that patients who were PMs at 2C19 responded better to omeprazole treatment for *Helicobacter pylori* gastritis, in terms of both amelioration of symptoms and eradication of *H. pylori.* This outcome is thought to be due to the higher exposure to serum omeprazole in PMs. The extensive metabolizers in the study had poorer outcomes at all dose ranges.

On the negative side, Chang et al. (1997) showed that the antitumor agents cyclophosphamide and ifosfamide are metabolized to their more active forms by 2C9 and 2C19. The drugs are also metabolized by 3A4. If a patient is a PM at either enzyme, his or her response to these agents may be compromised.

■ ARE THERE DRUGS THAT INHIBIT 2C19 ACTIVITY?

Yes. Fluvoxamine is a potent inhibitor of 2C19 (Rasmussen et al. 1998). Other inhibitors include the selective serotonin reuptake inhibitors paroxetine and fluoxetine (both less potent than fluvoxamine), ticlopidine (Donahue et al. 1999), modafinil (Grozinger et al. 1998; Provigil 1999), and omeprazole (Ko et al. 1997).

Fortunately, as mentioned previously, only a few drugs are selectively dependent on 2C19 for metabolism, so clinical inhibition is not usually a problem (except in the case of the drugs noted).

■ ARE THERE DRUGS THAT INDUCE 2C19 ACTIVITY?

Yes. Rifampin has been known to induce 2C19 as well as 2C9 (Zhou et al. 1990). However, there are no clinical reports of rifampin's decreasing serum levels of 2C19-dependent drugs.

■ REFERENCES

Aoyama N, Tanigawara Y, Kita T, et al: Sufficient effect of 1-week omeprazole and amoxicillin dual treatment for *Helicobacter pylori* eradication in cytochrome P450 2C19 poor metabolizers. J Gastroenterol 34 (suppl 11):80–83, 1999

Chang TK, Yu L, Goldstein JA, et al: Identification of the polymorphically expressed CYP2C19 and the wild-type CYP2C9-ILE359 allele as low-Km catalysts of cyclophosphamide and ifosfamide. Pharmacogenetics 7:211–221, 1997

Donahue S, Flockhart DA, Abernathy DR: Ticlopidine inhibits phenytoin clearance. Clin Pharmacol Ther 66:563–568, 1999

Flockhart DA: Drug interactions and the cytochrome P450 system: a role of cytochrome P450 2C19. Clin Pharmacokinet 29 (suppl 1):45–52, 1995

Glue P, Banfield CR, Perhach JL, et al: Pharmacokinetic interactions with felbamate: in vitro-in vivo correlation. Clin Pharmacokinet 33:214–224, 1997

Grozinger M, Hartter S, Hiemke C, et al: Interaction of modafinil and clomipramine as comedication in a narcoleptic patient. Clin Neuropharmacol 21:127–129, 1998

Jung F, Griffin KJ, Song W, et al: Identification of amino acid substitutions that confer a high affinity for sulfaphenazole binding and a high catalytic efficiency for warfarin metabolism to P450 2C19. Biochemistry 37:16270–16279, 1998

Kaneko A, Lum JK, Yaviong L, et al: High and variable frequencies of CYP2C19 mutations: medical consequences of poor metabolism in Vanuatu and other Pacific islands. Pharmacogenetics 9:581–590, 1999

Ko JW, Sukhova N, Thacker D, et al: Evaluation of omeprazole and lansoprazole as inhibitors of cytochrome P450 isoforms. Drug Metab Dispos 25:853–862, 1997

Provigil package insert. West Chester, PA, Cephalon, Inc, 1999

Rasmussen BB, Nielsen TL, Brosen K: Fluvoxamine inhibits the CYP2C19-catalysed metabolism of proguanil in vitro. Eur J Clin Pharmacol 54:735–740, 1998

Wedlund PJ, Aslanian WS, McAllister CB, et al: Mephenytoin hydroxylation deficiency in Caucasians: frequency of a new oxidative drug metabolism polymorphism. Clin Pharmacol Ther 36:773–780, 1984

Wrighton SA, Stevens JC, Becker GW, et al: Isolation and characterization of human liver cytochrome P450 2C19: a correlation between 2C19 and S-mephenytoin 4′-hydroxylation. Arch Biochem Biophys 306:240–245, 1993

Zhou HH, Anthony LB, Wood AJ, et al: Induction of polymorphic 4′-hydroxylation of S-mephenytoin by rifampicin. Br J Clin Pharmacol 30:471–475, 1990

■ STUDY CASE

A 42-year-old Caucasian man who had been on phenytoin 300 mg/day for 5 years for a seizure disorder was started on ticlopidine 250 mg po bid. Baseline routine phenytoin levels before starting ticlopidine ranged from 13 mg/L to 19 mg/L. Three days after starting ticlopidine, he reported dizziness and somnolence. A phenytoin level was checked and was in the toxic range of 44 mg/L.

Comment

2C19 inhibition by ticlopidine: Ticlopidine is a potent, specific inhibitor of 2C19. Phenytoin, although metabolized by 2C9 and phase II conjugation enzymes, is also metabolized by 2C19. There are many case reports of this particular interaction.

Reference

Donahue S, Flockhart DA, Abernathy DR: Ticlopidine inhibits phenytoin clearance. Clin Pharmacol Ther 66:563–568, 1999

■ DRUGS METABOLIZED BY 2C19

Antidepressants[1]	Barbiturates	Proton pump inhibitors	Other drugs
Amitriptyline	Hexobarbital	Lansoprazole[3]	Cilostazol
Citalopram	Mephobarbital	Omeprazole[3]	Cyclophosphamide[4]
Clomipramine		Pantoprazole[3]	Diazepam[5]
Imipramine		Rabeprazole[3]	Ifosfamide[4]
Moclobemide			Mephenytoin[2]
			Proguanil
			Propranolol
			Teniposide

[1]Tricyclic antidepressants and citalopram are metabolized by a variety of P450 enzymes.
[2]The isomer S-mephenytoin is used as a probe for 2C19 activity.
[3]Also metabolized by 3A4.
[4]Also metabolized by 3A4. However, this agent is a pro-drug that is activated by 2C19 enzyme activity.
[5]Also metabolized by other P450 enzymes.

■ INHIBITORS OF 2C19

Selective serotonin reuptake inhibitors	Other drugs
Fluoxetine[b]	Delavirdine
Fluvoxamine[a]	Felbamate
Paroxetine[c]	Ketoconazole
	Lansoprazole
	Modafinil
	Omeprazole[a]
	Ranitidine
	Ritonavir[a]
	Ticlopidine[a]

■ INDUCERS OF 2C19

Phenytoin[b]
Rifabutin
Rifapentine
Valproic acid

[a]Potent (bold type).
[b]Moderate.
[c]Mild.

9

2E1

2E1 is the least clinically important of the six enzymes described in this guide. However, there are a few clinically meaningful issues related to 2E1; they are discussed in this chapter.

■ WHAT DOES 2E1 DO?

2E1 is important in the metabolism of carcinogens and organic solvents. It also metabolizes some chemicals into carcinogens. Depending on its substrate, 2E1 may oxidize or reduce compounds (Koop 1992).

■ WHERE IS 2E1?

2E1 is found almost exclusively in the liver and accounts for about 5% of all cytochrome activity. The gene, like the genes of the 2C subfamily, is located on chromosome 10.

■ DOES 2E1 HAVE ANY POLYMORPHISMS?

Yes, but the significance of these polymorphisms is unclear. 2E1's link to carcinogenesis and even alcohol dependence has placed the polymorphisms of 2E1 under much scrutiny. Phenotypic variability of this enzyme carries many implications. For example, if compounds such as benzene and aniline (known carcinogens) are metabolized by 2E1, then having more or less activity may affect the risk of cancer. In addition, the application of bench research data to clinical practice is difficult. 2E1 activity is easily *induced* by alcohol consumption (Lieber 1997) and obesity (Kotlyar and Carson 1999). It is *inhibited* by disulfiram (Chick 1999) and even just one serving of watercress (Leclercq et al. 1998)! Determining the significance of being a poor metabolizer (PM), extensive metabolizer (EM), or ultraextensive metabolizer (UEM) at this enzyme is difficult in clinical practice (Carriere et al. 1996; Itoga et al. 1998). Although different alleles have been found in Mexican Americans (Wan et al. 1998), Japanese (Sun et al. 1999), and Caucasians (Grove et al. 1998), clinical conclusions regarding 2E1 polymorphisms should not be drawn at this time. The reader is encouraged to wait for more data.

■ ARE THERE DRUGS THAT INHIBIT 2E1 ACTIVITY?

Yes. Disulfiram may be the best-known inhibitor of 2E1. A single 500-mg dose of disulfiram significantly inhibits 2E1 activity up to 10 hours later (Kharasch et al. 1993). The drug's metabolite diethylcarbamate also inhibits 2E1. Disulfiram inhibits only 2E1, not the other P450 enzymes (Kharasch et al. 1999).

Isoniazid both inhibits and induces 2E1 (Zand et al. 1993). When treatment with isoniazid is initiated, the drug immediately inhibits 2E1 (competitive inhibition), increasing levels of other compounds dependent on 2E1 for metabolism. After isoniazid therapy has continued for several weeks, the drug decreases the serum levels of the same compounds. Induction by isoniazid may be the reason its use with acetaminophen is associated with hepatotoxicity (Self et al. 1999).

■ ARE THERE DRUGS THAT INDUCE 2E1 ACTIVITY?

Yes. The best-known inducer of 2E1 is ethyl alcohol (Seitz and Csomos 1992), used either acutely or chronically (Koop 1992). Alcohol can increase 2E1 activity 10-fold. Of course, alcohol has many other undesired effects on the liver (Lieber 1997).

The other inducers of 2E1 are isoniazid (which, as noted earlier, both inhibits and induces 2E1) and obesity (Kotlyar and Carson 1999). Obesity induces none of the other P450 enzymes besides 2E1; however, obesity appears to be associated with some decrease in function (by an unclear mechanism) of 3A4.

■ MISCELLANEOUS ISSUES

Chlorzoxazone (Parafon Forte), a skeletal muscle relaxant, is metabolized to 6-hydroxychlorzoxazone strictly by 2E1, which makes it an ideal probe for 2E1 activity to help identify poor metabolizers or drugs that inhibit or induce 2E1 (Lucas et al. 1999).

2E1's role in the metabolism of acetaminophen is minimal. When 2E1 metabolizes acetaminophen, however, the metabolite is hepatotoxic. In normal circumstances, the liver can quickly detoxify the metabolite. But if the usual hepatic metabolism of acetaminophen is overwhelmed, either by an acetaminophen overdose or by induction of 2E1 through chronic alcohol use (thereby increasing the percentage of acetaminophen being metabolized by 2E1), clinical hepatotoxic effects are possible. *N*-Acetylcysteine is used to avoid hepatotoxicity in cases of acetaminophen overdose. *N*-Acetylcysteine enhances glutathione conjugation in the liver, which enhances elimination of the toxic metabolite (Ziment 1988).

Alcoholic individuals have a higher risk of developing hepatotoxicity from therapeutic doses of acetaminophen (Seeff et al. 1986). Administration of 2E1 inhibitors (such as disulfiram or even watercress) to alcoholic patients might protect these patients from acetaminophen hepatotoxicity, but studies to date have been small or inconclusive (Poulsen et al. 1991).

■ REFERENCES

Carriere V, Berthou F, Baird S, et al: Human cytochrome P450 2E1 (CYP2E1): from genotype to phenotype. Pharmacogenetics 6:203–211, 1996

Chick J: Safety issues concerning the use of disulfiram in treating alcohol dependence. Drug Saf 20:427–435, 1999

Grove J, Brown AS, Daly AK, et al: The RsaI polymorphism of CYP2E1 and susceptibility to alcoholic liver disease in Caucasians: effect on age of presentation and dependence on alcohol dehydrogenase genotype. Pharmacogenetics 8:335–342, 1998

Itoga S, Harada S, Nomura F, et al: Genetic polymorphism of human CYP2E1: new alleles detected in exons and exon-intron junctions. Nihon Arukoru Yakubutsu Igakkai Zasshi 33:56–64, 1998

Kharasch ED, Thummel KE, Mhyre J, et al: Single-dose disulfiram inhibition of chlorzoxazone metabolism: a clinical probe for P450 2E1. Clin Pharmacol Ther 53:643–650, 1993

Kharasch ED, Hankins DC, Jubert C, et al: Lack of single-dose disulfiram effects on cytochrome P-450 2C9, 2C19, 2D6, and 3A4 activities: evidence for specificity toward P-450 2E1. Drug Metab Dispos 27:717–723, 1999

Koop DR: Oxidative and reductive metabolism by cytochrome P450 2E1. FASEB J 6:724–730, 1992

Kotlyar M, Carson SW: Effects of obesity on the cytochrome P450 enzyme system. Int J Clin Pharmacol Ther 37:8–19, 1999

Leclercq I, Desager JP, Horsmans Y: Inhibition of chlorzoxazone metabolism, a clinical probe for CYP2E1, by a single ingestion of watercress. Clin Pharmacol Ther 64:144–149, 1998

Lieber CS: Ethanol metabolism, cirrhosis and alcoholism. Clin Chim Acta 257:59–84, 1997

Lucas D, Ferrara R, Gonzalez E, et al: Chlorzoxazone, a selective probe for phenotyping CYP2E1 in humans. Pharmacogenetics 9:377–388, 1999

Poulsen HH, Ranek L, Jorgensen L: The influence of disulfiram on acetaminophen metabolism in man. Xenobiotica 21:243–249, 1991

Seeff LB, Cuccherini BA, Zimmerman HJ, et al: Acetaminophen hepatotoxicity in alcoholics: a therapeutic misadventure. Ann Intern Med 104:399–404, 1986

Seitz HK, Csomos G: Alcohol and the liver: ethanol metabolism and the pathomechanism of alcoholic liver damage [in Hungarian]. Orv Hetil 133:3183–3189, 1992

Self TH, Chrisman CR, Baciewicz AM, et al: Isoniazid drug and food interactions. Am J Med Sci 317:304–311, 1999

Sun F, Tsuritani I, Honda R, et al: Association of genetic polymorphisms of alcohol-metabolizing enzymes with excessive alcohol consumption in Japanese men. Hum Genet 105:295–300, 1999

Wan YJ, Poland RE, Lin KM: Genetic polymorphism of CYP2E1, ADH2, and ALDH2 in Mexican-Americans. Genet Test 2:79–83, 1998

Zand R, Nelson SD, Slattery JT, et al: Inhibition and induction of cytochrome P4502E1-catalyzed oxidation by isoniazid in humans. Clin Pharmacol Ther 54:142–149, 1993

Ziment I: Acetylcysteine: a drug that is much more than a mucokinetic. Biomed Pharmacother 42:513–519, 1988

■ STUDY CASE

A 26-year-old Caucasian man who had been binge drinking for several weeks decided to stop drinking. After 2 days of abstinence, he took five 650-mg tablets of acetaminophen. Forty-eight hours later he was brought to the emergency room with symptoms of hepatitis.

Comment

2E1 induction by ethanol: The patient's 2E1 enzymes were induced by the chronic, heavy ethanol consumption. When a large dose of acetaminophen is taken, the enhanced 2E1 enzymes metabolize acetaminophen into the hepatotoxic metabolite *N*-acetyl-*p*-benzoquinone imine (NAPQI). A theoretical therapeutic option is to give the patient a potent 2E1 inhibitor, such as disulfiram, to stop the metabolism of acetaminophen by 2E1.

Reference

Manyike PT, Kharasch ED, Kalhorn TF, et al: Contribution of CYP2E1 and CYP3A to acetaminophen reactive metabolite formation. Clin Pharmacol Ther 67:275–282, 2000

98

■ DRUGS METABOLIZED BY 2E1

Anesthetics	Other drugs
Enflurane	Acetaminophen[1]
Halothane	Aniline
Isoflurane	Benzene
	Carbon tetrachloride[2]
	Chlorzoxazone[3]
	Dacarbazine[2]
	Ethanol[4]
	Verapamil[5]

[1] Minor substrate, except in cases of overdose or induction of 2E1.
[2] Metabolism by 2E1 leads to production of a liver-toxic metabolite.
[3] Used as a probe for 2E1 activity.
[4] Metabolized by other hepatic and extrahepatic enzymes.
[5] Also metabolized by 3A4 and 2C9.

■ INHIBITORS OF 2E1

Chlormethiozole
Diethylcarbamate
Disulfiram
Isoniazid
Watercress

■ INDUCERS OF 2E1

Ethanol
Isoniazid
Obesity
Retinoids

PART III

P450 Considerations by Medical Specialty

GYNECOLOGY: ORAL CONTRACEPTIVES

Jessica R. Oesterheld, M.D.

Forty years ago, the introduction of Enovid (norethynodrel 10 mg and mestranol 150 μg), which provided convenient and reliable contraception, revolutionized birth control. Reports of interactions between oral contraceptives (OCs) and other drugs began to trickle into the literature. At first, these drug interactions appeared to be random and unrelated. Increased understanding of P450 enzymes and phase II reactions of sulfation and glucuronidation has permitted preliminary categorization and assessment of the clinical relevance of these drug interactions.

> Reminder: In this chapter, only P450-mediated interactions are discussed. Interactions due to displaced protein-binding, alterations in absorption or excretion, and pharmacodynamic interactions are not covered.

■ ORAL CONTRACEPTIVES

Most OCs contain both estrogen and progestin. The estrogen suppresses ovulation, and the progestin suppresses luteinizing hormone, to create an environment unreceptive to sperm. In addition,

Portions of this chapter are adapted from Shader RI, Oesterheld JR: "Contraceptive Effectiveness: Cytochromes and Induction." *Journal of Clinical Psychopharmacology* 20:119–121, 2000.

progestins limit endometrial hyperplasia and decrease the likelihood of endometrial carcinoma. There has been a strong trend in recent years toward using lower-dose estrogen preparations, to reduce the likelihood of estrogen-related complications (e.g., headache and thromboembolic disorders). Most OCs contain between 20 and 50 µg of estrogen, usually in the form of 17α-ethinylestradiol. Only a few OCs contain the original estrogen, mestranol, the 3-methyl ether of ethinyl estradiol (EE). Several formulations of OCs are available. Monophasic preparations contain the same amount of EE and progestin and are taken for 21 days in each 28-day cycle. Biphasic and triphasic preparations take the form of two or three types of pills, with varying amounts of active ingredients. Biphasic and triphasic OCs have been formulated so that the amount of progestin is reduced and the effects correspond more closely to hormonal influences during natural menstrual cycles. There are a limited number of progestin-only contraceptives. These contraceptives are the minipill, which contains 350 µg of norethindrone or 75 µg of norgestrel; a subdermal implant of norgestrel (Norplant); an intramuscular preparation of medroxyprogesterone acetate (Depo-Provera), given every 3 months; and an intrauterine device (Progestasert).

Metabolism of Oral Contraceptives

The metabolism of OCs is incompletely understood. Mestranol is first metabolized by 2C9 to EE. After first-pass metabolism, about half of EE reaches the systemic circulation unchanged; the remainder is metabolized in the liver and gut wall. Although a variety of metabolic pathways exist (including sulfation in the gut wall), the major route of inactivation of EE is via 3A4 (Guengerich 1990b). An enterohepatic recirculation is also postulated for conjugated EE (but is not important for progestins). EE is hydrolyzed by gut bacteria (principally clostridia) back to free EE. Further metabolic steps include catechol oxidation and glucuronidation via glucuronosyltransferase 1A1, the same isoform responsible for glucuronidation of bilirubin.

3A4 Induction of Oral Contraceptives

Induction of 3A4 may lead to increased clearance of EE and/or progestins and loss of clinical efficacy. Drug interactions resulting in spotting, breakthrough bleeding, or unwanted pregnancy have occurred in women taking OCs and griseofulvin (van Dijke and Weber 1984), ritonavir (chronic use [Ouellet et al. 1998]), rifampin (Joshi et al. 1980), troglitazone (Loi et al. 1999), or enzyme-inducing anticonvulsants (phenobarbital, primidone, phenytoin [Baciewicz 1985], or oxcarbazepine [Fattore et al. 1999]). Carbamazepine can both render OCs ineffective and cause fetal neural tube defects. Topiramate and felbamate may also induce 3A4. These two drugs increase clearance of EE (Rosenfeld et al. 1997; Saano et al. 1995), and it is possible that they also cause contraceptive failure. A combination HIV drug, a protease inhibitor containing lopinavir and ritonavir, carries a manufacturer's warning about lopinavir/ritonavir's ability to induce metabolism of EE. This drug induces glucuronidation and may also induce metabolism of EE at 3A4 (Abbott Laboratories, Products Division personal communication, December 2000). St. John's wort has recently been shown to induce 3A4 through activation of the pregnane receptor (Moore et al. 2000; Roby et al. 2000), and the herbal preparation is likely to cause contraceptive failure, although formal case reports have not yet entered the literature. Clinicians should ask their patients about use of St. John's wort. Some anticonvulsants/mood stabilizers (valproate [Crawford et al. 1986], gabapentin [Eldon et al. 1998], lamotrigine [Holdich et al. 1991; Hussein and Posner 1997], and vigabatrin [Bartoli et al. 1997]) have been shown *not* to increase OC clearance.

3A4 inducers also increase clearance of progestin-only contraceptives, substrates (metabolites) of 3A4. Although not as well documented as interactions involving EE, contraceptive failure of levonorgestrel has been reported in women given phenobarbital (Shane-McWhorter et al. 1998) and phenytoin (Haukkamaa 1986; Odlind and Olsson 1986).

There are reports of women becoming pregnant while taking both EE or progestin-only preparations and other drugs, but it is not known how common such pregnancies are. Pharmacokinetic inter-

■ SUBSTANCES THAT INTERACT WITH ORAL CONTRACEPTIVES

Some drugs and herbal preparations that induce 3A4 and can cause contraceptive failure	Some drugs and foods that may increase or prolong oral contraceptive activity	Drugs whose clearance is decreased by oral contraceptives
Carbamazepine	Acetaminophen	Amitriptyline
Felbamate	Antifungals: fluconazole,	Caffeine
Griseofulvin	ketoconazole, itraconazole	Chlordiazepoxide
Oxcarbazepine	Erythromycin, other macrolides	?Clozapine
Phenobarbital	Fluoxetine	?Cox-2 inhibitors
Phenytoin	Fluvoxamine	Cyclosporine
Primidone	?Gestodene	Diazepam
Rifampin	Grapefruit juice	Imipramine
Ritonavir	Nefazodone	?Olanzapine
St. John's wort	Ritonavir	Phenytoin
Topiramate	Vitamin C	Prednisolone
Troglitazone		?Proton pump inhibitors
		Selegiline
		?Tacrine
		Theophylline

? = unknown.

actions between OCs and 3A4 inducers do occur, but how often do
clinically significant pharmacodynamic outcomes result? Given the
wide interindividual variation of 3A4, some women may be vulnerable to these drug interactions. A recent small clinical study of
rifampin, rifabutin, and OCs substantiated the ability of rifampin
and rifabutin to increase clearance of OCs, although none of the
12 women in the study ovulated (Barditch-Crovo et al. 1999). Currently, lower and lower dosing of EE is being used, and women who
take these minidoses may be especially vulnerable. It is recommended that until clinicians can identify women at risk, patients
taking enzyme-inducing anticonvulsants (except phenytoin [see the
discussion later in this chapter]) with OCs take the former with 50–
100 µg of EE. Another option is more frequent dosing of intramuscular preparations of progestin-only OCs. In addition to either of
these approaches, women taking enzyme-inducing drugs along
with OCs should also be instructed to use barrier contraceptives
midcycle, to prevent pregnancy (Crawford et al. 1990). Replacement of 3A4-inducing anticonvulsants with noninducing alterna-
tives should also be considered (Guberman 1999). An enzyme
inducer's effects can continue after administration of the inducer
has ceased. As has been recommended with rifampin use ("Use of
Rifampin and Contraceptive Steroids" 1999), after short-term treatment with 3A4 inducers is discontinued, patients taking OCs need
to take extra contraceptive precautions for up to 4 weeks.

3A4 Inhibition of Oral Contraceptives

Because EE is a 3A4 substrate, potent inhibitors of 3A4 can decrease EE clearance and increase or prolong estrogenic activity. Although not likely to impair contraceptive efficacy, potent 3A4
inhibitors can be expected to increase estrogen-related side effects
(e.g., migraine headaches or thromboembolic events) in susceptible
women. Well-described drugs known to increase EE levels include
the antifungals ketoconazole, itraconazole, and fluconazole (Sinofsky and Pasquale 1998); antivirals such as ritonavir; and potent
macrolides (Meyer et al. 1990; Pessayre 1983; Wermeling et al.
1995). Even grapefruit juice is known to increase EE levels (Weber

et al. 1996). Although gestodene has been shown to increase EE in vitro (Guengerich 1990a), this interaction may not be clinically significant (Lawrenson and Farmer 2000). It is likely that psychotropics (e.g., nefazodone, fluvoxamine, and fluoxetine) known to potently inhibit 3A4 will also be shown to affect EE clearance. EE clearance also decreases when vitamin C or acetaminophen is added. This interaction between EE and vitamin C or acetaminophen is noncytochromal but occurs because both agents compete for sulfation with EE in the gut wall (Rogers et al. 1987).

Mestranol is demethylated to EE by 2C9, so potent inhibitors of 2C9 may lessen the likelihood of adequate EE levels. Examples of 2C9 inhibitors are sulfaphenazole and other sulfonamide antibiotics and the psychotropics fluvoxamine and valproate. Once demethylated, mestranol is as susceptible to induction or inhibition as any EE.

1A2, 2C19, and 3A4 Inhibition by Oral Contraceptives

Not only is clearance of OCs affected by other agents, but OCs can affect clearance of other drugs. Current evidence suggests that OCs are moderate inhibitors of 1A2 and 2C19 and modest or mild inhibitors of 3A4. OCs decrease clearance of caffeine and theophylline, well-known substrates of 1A2 (Abernethy and Todd 1985; Gu et al. 1992; Roberts et al. 1983; Tornatore et al. 1982; Zhang and Kaminsky 1995). Because a 30% decrease in theophylline clearance occurs with OC use (Jonkman 1986), clinicians should decrease theophylline doses. Although the side-chain oxidation of propranolol is a 1A2 phenomenon (Yoshimoto et al. 1995) and is inhibited by OCs (Walle et al. 1996), because of nullifying effects of OCs on propranolol glucuronidation no significant interaction occurs (Walle et al. 1989; Walle et al. 1996). No reports of interactions between OCs and the psychotropic 1A2 substrates olanzapine, clozapine, and tacrine are currently found in the literature, although these drug interactions are possible. Plasma concentrations of tacrine have been shown to be increased by hormone replacement therapy (HRT) (Laine et al. 1999) and are likely increased by OCs.

Additional support for OCs' inhibition of 2C19 was provided by two recent population studies (Laine et al. 2000; Tamminga et al. 1999). The activity of 2C19 in women who used OCs was decreased by 68% compared with that in women who did not use OCs (Tamminga et al. 1999). Although the focus of interest in the OC-phenytoin interaction has been on phenytoin's induction of OC metabolism, OCs have also been found to decrease clearance of phenytoin (De Leacy et al. 1979). Thus, increasing OC dosing to overcome phenytoin induction of EE can result in phenytoin toxicity, and this drug combination is best avoided. No information regarding other 2C19 substrates (e.g., proton pump inhibitors or cyclooxygenase-2 inhibitors) was found, but these drugs may be similarly affected.

Head-to-head in vitro comparisons of EE and gestodene have shown EE to be an inhibitor of 3A4, but EE is not as potent as gestodene (Guengerich 1990a). There is less evidence to support EE's in vivo 3A4 inhibition. Although concentrations of EE are higher in women who take OCs for more than 6 months, clearance of EE in these women is reduced (Tornatore et al. 1982). Other inferential evidence comes from several interactions between OCs and drugs known to be substrates of 3A4: cyclosporine (Deray et al. 1987), prednisolone (Seidegard et al. 2000), and levonorgestrel (Fotherby 1991).

Inhibition by OCs of both 3A4 and 2C19 is likely responsible for several well-documented OC-drug interactions. Clearances of imipramine, amitriptyline, and diazepam are decreased by OCs (Abernethy et al. 1982, 1984; Edelbroek et al. 1987). 2C19 is the principal pathway for demethylation of these drugs; 3A4 is also involved (Jung et al. 1997; Koyama et al. 1997; Venkatakrishnan et al. 1998). Clearance of chlordiazepoxide may also be reduced by OCs (Patwardhan et al. 1983). Chlordiazepoxide's intermediate metabolite, nordiazepam, is known to be metabolized by 3A4 and 2C19 (Ono et al. 1996). Whether other benzodiazepines that are metabolized via this intermediate metabolite are also affected has not yet been investigated.

■ REFERENCES

Abernethy DR, Todd EL: Impairment of caffeine clearance by chronic use of low-dose oestrogen-containing oral contraceptives. Eur J Clin Pharmacol 28:425–428, 1985

Abernethy DR, Greenblatt DJ, Divoll M, et al: Impairment of diazepam metabolism by low-dose estrogen-containing oral-contraceptive steroids. N Engl J Med 306:791–792, 1982

Abernethy DR, Greenblatt DJ, Shader RI: Imipramine disposition in users of oral contraceptive steroids. Clin Pharmacol Ther 35:792–797, 1984

Baciewicz AM: Oral contraceptive drug interactions. Ther Drug Monit 7:26–35, 1985

Barditch-Crovo P, Trapnell CB, Ette E, et al: The effects of rifampin and rifabutin on the pharmacokinetics and pharmacodynamics of a combination oral contraceptive. Clin Pharmacol Ther 65:428–438, 1999

Bartoli A, Gatti G, Cipolla G, et al: A double-blind, placebo-controlled study on the effect of vigabatrin on in vivo parameters of hepatic microsomal enzyme induction and on the kinetics of steroid oral contraceptives in healthy female volunteers. Epilepsia 38:702–707, 1997

Crawford P, Chadwick D, Cleland P, et al: The lack of effect of sodium valproate on the pharmacokinetics of oral contraceptive steroids. Contraception 33:23–29, 1986

Crawford P, Chadwick DJ, Martin C, et al: The interaction of phenytoin and carbamazepine with combined oral contraceptive steroids. Br J Clin Pharmacol 30:892–896, 1990

De Leacy EA, McLeay CD, Eadie MJ, et al: Effects of subjects' sex, and intake of tobacco, alcohol and oral contraceptives on plasma phenytoin levels. Br J Clin Pharmacol 8:33–36, 1979

Deray G, le Hoang P, Cacoub P, et al: Oral contraceptive interaction with cyclosporin. Lancet 1:158–159, 1987

Edelbroek PM, Zitman FG, Knoppert-van der Klein EA, et al: Therapeutic drug monitoring of amitriptyline: impact of age, smoking and contraceptives on drug and metabolite levels in bulimic women. Clin Chim Acta 165:177–187, 1987

Eldon MA, Underwood BA, Randinitis EJ, et al: Gabapentin does not interact with a contraceptive regimen of norethindrone acetate and ethinyl estradiol. Neurology 50:1146–1148, 1998

Fattore C, Cipolla G, Gatti G, et al: Induction of ethinylestradiol and levonorgestrel metabolism by oxcarbazepine in healthy women. Epilepsia 40:783–787, 1999

Fotherby K: Intrasubject variability in the pharmacokinetics of ethynyl-oestradiol. J Steroid Biochem Mol Biol 38:733–736, 1991

Gu L, Gonzalez FJ, Kalow W, et al: Biotransformation of caffeine, paraxanthine, theobromine and theophylline by cDNA-expressed human CYP1A2 and CYP2E1. Pharmacogenetics 2:73–77, 1992

Guberman A: Hormonal contraception and epilepsy. Neurology 53 (suppl 1):838–840, 1999

Guengerich FP: Inhibition of oral contraceptive steroid-metabolizing enzymes by steroids and drugs. Am J Obstet Gynecol 163:2159–2163, 1990a

Guengerich FP: Metabolism of 17 alpha-ethynylestradiol in humans. Life Sci 47:1981–1988, 1990b

Haukkamaa M: Contraception by Norplant subdermal capsules is not reliable in epileptic patients on anticonvulsant treatment. Contraception 33:559–565, 1986

Holdich T, Whiteman P, Orme M, et al: Effect of lamotrigine on the pharmacology of the combined oral contraceptive pill (abstract). Epilepsia 32 (suppl 1):96, 1991

Hussein Z, Posner J: Population pharmacokinetics of lamotrigine monotherapy in patients with epilepsy: retrospective analysis of routine monitoring data. Br J Clin Pharmacol 43:457–465, 1997

Jonkman JH: Therapeutic consequences of drug interactions with theophylline pharmacokinetics. J Allergy Clin Immunol 78:736–742, 1986

Joshi JV, Joshi UM, Sankolli GM, et al: A study of interactions of a low-dose combination oral contraceptive with anti-tubercular drugs. Contraception 21:617–629, 1980

Jung F, Richardson TH, Raucy JL, et al: Diazepam metabolism by cDNA-expressed human 2C P450s: identification of P4502C18 and P4502C19 as low K(M) diazepam N-demethylases. Drug Metab Dispos 25:133–139, 1997

Koyama E, Chiba K, Tani M, et al: Reappraisal of human CYP isoforms involved in imipramine N-demethylation and 2-hydroxylation: a study using microsomes obtained from putative extensive and poor metabolizers of S-mephenytoin and eleven recombinant human CYPs. J Pharmacol Exp Ther 281:1199–1210, 1997

Laine K, Palovaara S, Tapanainen P, et al: Plasma tacrine concentrations are significantly increased by concomitant hormone replacement therapy. Clin Pharmacol Ther 66:602–608, 1999

Laine K, Tybring G, Bertilsson L: No sex-related differences but significant inhibition by oral contraceptives of CYP2C19 activity as measured by the probe drugs mephenytoin and omeprazole in healthy Swedish white subjects. Clin Pharmacol Ther 68:151–159, 2000

Lawrenson R, Farmer R: Venous thromboembolism and combined oral contraceptives: does the type of progestogen make a difference? Contraception 62 (suppl 2):S21–S28, 2000

Loi CM, Stern R, Koup JR, et al: Effect of troglitazone on the pharmacokinetics of an oral contraceptive agent. J Clin Pharmacol 39:410–417, 1999

Meyer B, Muller F, Wessels P, et al: A model to detect interactions between roxithromycin and oral contraceptives. Clin Pharmacol Ther 47:671–674, 1990

Moore LB, Goodwin B, Jones SA, et al: St. John's wort induces hepatic drug metabolism through activation of the pregnane X receptor. Proc Natl Acad Sci U S A 97:7500–7502, 2000

Odlind V, Olsson SE: Enhanced metabolism of levonorgestrel during phenytoin treatment in a woman with Norplant implants. Contraception 33:257–261, 1986

Ono S, Hatanaka T, Miyazawa S, et al: Human liver microsomal diazepam metabolism using cDNA-expressed cytochrome P450s: role of CYP2B6, 2C19 and the 3A subfamily. Xenobiotica 26:1155–1166, 1996

Ouellet D, Hsu A, Qian J, et al: Effect of ritonavir on the pharmacokinetics of ethinyl oestradiol in healthy female volunteers. Br J Clin Pharmacol 46:111–116, 1998

Patwardhan RV, Mitchell MC, Johnson RF, et al: Differential effects of oral contraceptive steroids on the metabolism of benzodiazepines. Hepatology 3:248–253, 1983

Pessayre D: Effects of macrolide antibiotics on drug metabolism in rats and in humans. Int J Clin Pharmacol Res 3:449–458, 1983

Roberts RK, Grice J, McGuffie C, et al: Oral contraceptive steroids impair the elimination of theophylline. J Lab Clin Med 101:821–825, 1983

Roby CA, Anderson GD, Kantor E, et al: St John's wort: effect on CYP3A4 activity. Clin Pharmacol Ther 67:451–457, 2000

Rogers SM, Back DJ, Stevenson PJ, et al: Paracetamol interaction with oral contraceptive steroids: increased plasma concentrations of ethinyloestradiol. Br J Clin Pharmacol 23:721–725, 1987

Rosenfeld WE, Doose DR, Walker SA, et al: Effect of topiramate on the pharmacokinetics of an oral contraceptive containing norethindrone and ethinyl estradiol in patients with epilepsy. Epilepsia 38:317–323, 1997

Saano V, Glue P, Banfield CR, et al: Effects of felbamate on the pharmacokinetics of a low-dose combination oral contraceptive. Clin Pharmacol Ther 58:523–531, 1995

Seidegard J, Simonsson M, Edsbacker S: Effect of an oral contraceptive on the plasma levels of budesonide and prednisolone and the influence on plasma cortisol. Clin Pharmacol Ther 67:373–381, 2000

Shane-McWhorter L, Cerveny JD, MacFarlane LL, et al: Enhanced metabolism of levonorgestrel during phenobarbital treatment and resultant pregnancy. Pharmacotherapy 18:1360–1364, 1998

Sinofsky FE, Pasquale SA: The effect of fluconazole on circulating ethinyl estradiol levels in women taking oral contraceptives. Am J Obstet Gynecol 178:300–304, 1998

Tamminga WJ, Wemer J, Oosterhuis B, et al: CYP2D6 and CYP2C19 activity in a large population of Dutch healthy volunteers: indications for oral contraceptive-related gender differences. Eur J Clin Pharmacol 55:177–184, 1999

Tornatore KM, Kanarkowski R, McCarthy TL, et al: Effect of chronic oral contraceptive steroids on theophylline disposition. Eur J Clin Pharmacol 23:129–134, 1982

Use of rifampin and contraceptive steroids. Br J Fam Plann 24:169–170, 1999

van Dijke CP, Weber JC: Interaction between oral contraceptives and griseofulvin. British Medical Journal (Clinical Research Edition) 288:1125–1126, 1984

Venkatakrishnan K, Greenblatt DJ, von Moltke LL, et al: Five distinct human cytochromes mediate amitriptyline N-demethylation in vitro: dominance of CYP 2C19 and 3A4. J Clin Pharmacol 38:112–121, 1998

Walle T, Walle UK, Cowart TD, et al: Pathway-selective sex differences in the metabolic clearance of propranolol in human subjects. Clin Pharmacol Ther 46:257–263, 1989

Walle T, Fagan TC, Walle UK, et al: Stimulatory as well as inhibitory effects of ethinyloestradiol on the metabolic clearances of propranolol in young women. Br J Clin Pharmacol 41:305–309, 1996

Weber A, Jager R, Borner A, et al: Can grapefruit juice influence ethinyl-estradiol bioavailability? Contraception 53:41–47, 1996

Wermeling DP, Chandler MH, Sides GD, et al: Dirithromycin increases ethinyl estradiol clearance without allowing ovulation. Obstet Gynecol 86:78–84, 1995

Yoshimoto K, Echizen H, Chiba K, et al: Identification of human CYP isoforms involved in the metabolism of propranolol enantiomers—N-desisopropylation is mediated mainly by CYP1A2. Br J Clin Pharmacol 39:421–431, 1995

Zhang Z-Y, Kaminsky LS: Characterization of human cytochromes P450 involved in theophylline 8-hydroxylation. Biochem Pharmacol 50:205–211, 1995

11

INTERNAL MEDICINE

A complete discussion of drugs used in general medicine would be impossible in this Concise Guide, and in fact, most drugs have not been fully studied. This chapter contains an in-depth examination of drugs that affect other drugs (i.e., inhibit or induce the metabolism of other drugs), along with some discussion of the P450 metabolic sites for drugs with narrow therapeutic windows.

We discuss cardiovascular drugs (antiarrhythmics, anticoagulants, antihyperlipidemics [hydroxymethylglutaryl–coenzyme A (HMG-CoA) reductase inhibitors], calcium-channel blockers [CCBs], and β-blockers), gastrointestinal drugs, and antidiabetic agents. Antimicrobials, which are used across medical and surgical specialties and produce the greatest number of P450-mediated drug interactions, have earned their own chapter (Chapter 12). Analgesics are covered in Chapter 15. We open the chapter with a historical review of allergy medications, the drugs where the quest for more information about the P450 system really began.

> Reminder: In this chapter, only P450-mediated interactions are discussed. Interactions due to displaced protein-binding, alterations in absorption or excretion, and pharmacodynamic interactions are not covered.

■ ALLERGY DRUGS

The specialty of allergy and immunology involves management of some of the world's most frequent ailments: allergic rhinitis or hay fever and asthma. Antihistamines are among the most widely prescribed medications in the world (Woosley 1996). Theophylline is still a common element in the treatment of asthma and chronic obstructive pulmonary disease, and its sensitivity to being inhibited by other drugs has made it an important tool in the study of drug interactions as a probe drug (see Chapter 3). Many of the toxic nonsedating antihistamines have been removed from the market or reformulated. Here, a review of allergy medications past and present serves as a way to discuss how our understanding of drug-drug interactions developed.

Histamine, Subtype 1 (H_1), Receptor Blockers and Leukotriene D_4/E_4 Receptor Antagonists

3A4 Inhibition of H_1 Receptor Antagonists

Drug interactions involving second-generation histamine, subtype 1 (H_1), receptor antagonists (or nonsedating antihistamines) were one of the first-studied drug-drug interactions relating to the P450 system. (Interactions involving fluoxetine and tricyclic antidepressants were noted earlier but were not associated with lethal or severe arrhythmias.) These newer antihistamines do not cross the blood-brain barrier and are more H_1 selective than the older drugs, resulting in less sedation, less weight gain, and fewer other antihistaminic side effects. The first report of life-threatening cardiac arrhythmia associated with the use of terfenadine appeared in 1989, when a patient developed an arrhythmia after an intentional overdose (Davies et al. 1989). Monahan et al. (1990) wrote the first article on the cause of an arrhythmia in conjunction with terfenadine therapy. A woman taking terfenadine and cefaclor developed *Candida* vaginitis and treated herself with ketoconazole that she had remaining from treatment of a previous episode of vaginitis. She developed palpitations and later torsades de pointes, even though she was taking standard doses of all medications. These case reports led to in vivo studies involving healthy volunteers, which clearly demonstrated that the potent 3A4 inhibitor ketoconazole increases levels of unmetabolized terfenadine and is associated with QT interval prolongation (Woosley 1996; Yap and Camm 1999).

■ ALLERGY DRUGS

Drug	Metabolism site(s)	Enzyme(s) inhibited
H₁-receptor antagonists		
Astemizole[1,2]	3A4[1]	None known
Cetirizine	None	None known
Ebastine[1]	3A4[1]	None known
Fexofenadine[3]	None	None known
Loratadine	3A4	None known
Terfenadine[1,2]	3A4[1]	None known
Leukotriene D₄/E₄ receptor antagonists		
Montelukast	3A4, 2C9	None known
Zafirlukast	2C9	2C9, 3A4, 1A2
Xanthines		
Theophylline	1A2	None known

[1] Arrhythmogenic parent compounds.
[2] No longer marketed in the United States.
[3] Active metabolite of terfenadine.

Terfenadine is a pro-drug that usually undergoes a rapid and nearly complete first-pass hepatic biotransformation, producing the active metabolite at 3A4. The parent or pro-drug is cardiotoxic in overdose or when its first-pass metabolism is impaired by another compound at the same hepatic enzyme (in this case, 3A4), causing prolongation of the QT interval. Terfenadine seems to block potassium channels and to be as potent as quinidine in inhibiting the delayed rectifier potassium channel in cardiac tissue (Yap and Camm 1999). Carboxyterfenadine (fexofenadine), terfenadine's active metabolite, is not cardiotoxic and has no known hepatic metabolism (it is eliminated unchanged in the urine). Terfenadine was sold over the counter for a time. The pro-drug terfenadine has been voluntarily removed by the manufacturer from the United States market and has been replaced by fexofenadine. Astemizole (which has also been taken off the United States market) and ebastine (which is available in Europe) also are arrhythmogenic at high doses, and this effect may be heightened when either of these drugs is administered with potent inhibitors of 3A4, including nefazodone, cyclosporine, some macrolide antibiotics, azole antifungals, antiretrovirals, selective serotonin reuptake inhibitors (SSRIs), and grapefruit juice (Renwick 1999; Slater et al. 1999; Woosley 1996; Yap and Camm 1999) (see "Allergy Drugs" table and Chapter 5).

Cetirizine is the carboxylic acid metabolite of hydroxyzine. With regard to cetirizine, there are no reports in the literature of QT prolongation or hepatic metabolism. In studies in which healthy volunteers were administered cetirizine at three times the recommended dose, no effect on QT interval was found. Loratadine is hepatically metabolized at 3A4 and 2D6 but is not associated with QT interval prolongation at high doses, even in in vivo drug interaction studies involving potent 3A4 inhibitors such as erythromycin (Woosley 1996; Yap and Camm 1999). Ebastine is also cardiotoxic at high doses and at time of publication is being considered for release in the United States.

1A2 Inhibition by Leukotriene D_4/E_4 Receptor Antagonists

Zafirlukast is a leukotriene D_4/E_4 receptor antagonist and is used in prophylactic and chronic treatment of asthma. This drug antagonizes the contractile activity of leukotrienes. Zafirlukast suppresses airway responses to antigens such as pollen and cat dander and inhibits bronchoconstriction. It is a moderate inhibitor of 2C9, 1A2, and possibly 3A4. In one case, zafirlukast's activity at 1A2 was implicated in increasing serum theophylline levels. The agent has also been reported to increase the half-life of warfarin (Katial et al. 1998). In vitro studies of montelukast do not reveal this leukotriene D_4/E_4 receptor antagonist to be an inhibitor or inducer, but it is metabolized at 3A4 and 2C9. Clinical studies of montelukast are under way. At time of publication, montelukast had been studied in healthy volunteers with warfarin (Van Hecken et al. 1999) and digoxin (Depre et al. 1999). No significant interactions with these two drugs were noted.

Summary

The nonsedating antihistamines with cardiotoxic parent drugs include terfenadine, astemizole, and ebastine, which in overdose or when inhibited by other compounds at the 3A4 enzyme may lead to palpitations, syncope, or fatal arrhythmias. None of the H_1-receptor antagonist nonsedating antihistamines are inhibitors or inducers in the P450 system. Zafirlukast does inhibit several enzymes in vitro, and there are case reports of interactions involving warfarin and theophylline via 1A2 inhibition.

Xanthines

Aminophylline and its active metabolite theophylline are thought to cause bronchodilation, or smooth muscle relaxation, and suppression of airway response to antigens or irritants in asthmatic patients. Clinical efficacy is achieved at serum levels of 5–20 µg/mL. Serum concentrations greater than 20 µg/mL produce adverse reactions, including nausea, vomiting, headache, tremor, seizures, cardiac arrhythmias, and death. With such a narrow therapeutic window and such dangerous toxic adverse reactions, this hepatically metabolized compound is very susceptible to drug interactions.

Theophylline is known to be metabolized at 1A2. Inhibitors of 1A2 therefore have the potential to increase serum theophylline levels (see Chapter 6). Serum levels of theophylline also may be decreased by compounds that induce 1A2, such as omeprazole, rifampin, caffeine, cigarette smoke, and some foods (see Chapter 6). Some metabolism of theophylline occurs at 2E1 (Rasmussen et al. 1997). Because theophylline metabolism is so sensitive to inhibition and induction and theophylline levels are easily measured, the drug is used as a probe in determining whether other compounds are metabolized at 1A2.

Upton (1991) reviewed the pharmacokinetic interactions of theophylline. He noted that in the 1980s, numerous investigators reported theophylline toxicity when the drug was administered with fluoroquinolones and quinolones and that rifampicin, carbamazepine, phenytoin, and barbiturates cause an increase in theophylline clearance, leading to subtherapeutic serum levels. Reports began appearing in 1991 of cases of theophylline toxicity when the agent was administered with fluvoxamine (Rasmussen et al. 1995). By the mid-1990s, it had been established, through in vitro human liver microsomal studies as well as in vivo healthy volunteer pharmacokinetic studies, that theophylline is inhibited at 1A2 by fluvoxamine and most fluoroquinolones (Batty et al. 1995). Despite these findings, and warnings in package inserts, cases of theophylline toxicity are still reported. Andrews (1998) reported a case of theophylline toxicity in which ciprofloxacin was added to an asthmatic patient's regimen to treat productive cough and resulted in hospitalization and hemodialysis. DeVane et al. (1997) reported that a patient at a residential-care facility who was being treated with fluvoxamine for depression with psychotic features was prescribed theophylline for chronic obstructive pulmonary disease by her primary care physician. The woman experienced confusion, lack of energy, reduced sleep, and nausea and vomiting, all leading to an acute hospital admission. The half-life of theophylline in this case was increased fivefold.

Zevin and Benowitz (1999), in their thorough review of tobacco smoking, reported on the effect of polycyclic hydrocarbons in tobacco smoke, which induce 1A2 and 2E1 and may result in a reduction of serum theophylline levels.

Summary

Theophylline is metabolized almost exclusively at 1A2 and has a narrow therapeutic index. Therefore, whenever possible, use of potent inhibitors of 1A2 (which include the fluoroquinolones [ciprofloxacin is the most potent] and the SSRI fluvoxamine) should be avoided. If it is necessary to administer a fluoroquinolone, the least-potent drug of that class must be chosen, and serum theophylline levels must be monitored (some clinicians suggest decreasing the theophylline daily dose by two-thirds).

■ CARDIOVASCULAR AGENTS

Antiarrhythmics

General Drug Interactions

2D6 inhibition *by* antiarrhythmics. Quinidine is associated with multiple drug interactions of significance. Quinidine is not a substrate for 2D6 (not metabolized by 2D6); rather, it is a potent inhibitor of 2D6. Full inhibition of the enzyme occurs when just one-sixth of the usual antiarrhythmic dose is given. Briefly, quinidine's potent inhibition of 2D6 means that mexiletine, flecainide, propafenone, tricyclic antidepressant, haloperidol, codeine, propranolol, or nifedipine toxicity may occur when quinidine is coadministered. Quinidine's stereoisomer, quinine, is not an inhibitor of 2D6. (For an excellent review of this drug and a full table with references to pertinent literature, see Grace and Camm 1998.) Note that quinidine's metabolism is at 3A4. Inhibition at this site by drugs such as nefazodone, erythromycin, astemizole, ketoconazole, ritonavir, or clarithromycin may lead to quinidine toxicity.

2D6 inhibition *of* antiarrhythmics. Mexiletine, encainide, and propafenone metabolism may be affected if a patient is administered a potent 2D6 inhibitor. When propafenone is coadministered with quinidine, propafenone toxicity may result, in the form of bradycardia, heart block, heart failure, or worsening arrhythmia

122

■ ANTIARRHYTHMICS

Drug	Metabolism site(s)	Enzyme(s) inhibited	Enzyme(s) induced
Flecainide[1]	2D6	None known	None known
Encainide	2D6	None known	None known
Lidocaine	3A4	1A2[c]	None known
Mexiletine[1]	2D6, 1A2	**1A2**[a]	1A2
Moricizine[2]	None known	None known	None known
Propafenone	2D6, 3A4	**1A2**[a]	None known
Quinidine	3A4	**2D6**[a]	None known
Tocainide	None known	1A2[c]	None known

[1]Also significant renal metabolism and elimination.
[2]Induces antipyrine metabolism and its own metabolism.

[a]Potent (bold type).
[b]Moderate.
[c]Mild.

(Morike and Roden 1994). Other potent 2D6 inhibitors include the SSRIs, cimetidine, and ritonavir.

1A2 inhibition by antiarrhythmics. Mexiletine and propafenone are potent 1A2 inhibitors and therefore may increase levels of theophylline, caffeine, warfarin (Kobayashi et al. 1998; Spinler et al. 1993; Wei et al. 1999), and potentially tacrine.

Induction by antiarrhythmics. Moricizine seems to induce its own metabolism and has been found to induce the metabolism of theophylline, diltiazem, and the probe antipyrine (Benedek et al. 1994; Pieniaszek et al. 1993; Shum et al. 1996). These findings may indicate that moricizine is a "pan-inducer," given the fact that 1A2, 3A4, and possibly 2D6 were induced. No other studies (including human liver microsomal studies or other probe studies of this drug) were found that indicated whether cytochrome induction or some other type of drug interaction occurs.

Psychotropic Drug Interactions

Tricyclic antidepressants. Antiarrhythmics should rarely be prescribed with tricyclic antidepressants, given tricyclic antidepressants' quinidine-like potential to prolong the QTc interval, as well as the potential for sudden death in postmyocardial infarction patients. Secondary amine tricyclics are metabolized at 2D6.

Haloperidol and clozapine. 2D6 is a metabolic site for haloperidol and clozapine, albeit a minor site for clozapine.

Olanzapine. Olanzapine is 30%–40% metabolized at 1A2. Therefore, if the drug is administered with 1A2 inhibitors, side effects of olanzapine may worsen.

Summary

The effectiveness of antiarrhythmics and the morbidity and mortality associated with their administration vary across patient groups, and very narrow therapeutic windows make drug interactions all the more tricky to predict. Buchert and Woosley (1992) carefully reviewed patient variability with regard to response to this group of drugs, as well as the genetically determined differences in metabolism. 2D6 and its genetic polymorphism have played roles in many of the untoward effects of these drugs. Mexiletine and propafenone are potent inhibitors of 1A2, and caution should be used when these drugs are administered with 1A2-dependent drugs such as theophylline, tacrine, and caffeine. (For an excellent review of CCBs, see Abernethy and Schwartz 1999.)

Anticoagulants

Warfarin is primarily metabolized at 2C9, with some contribution from 2C19, 2C8, 2C18, 1A2, and 3A4. The *S*-enantiomer of warfarin is metabolized at 2C9 and is the more active isomer. *R*-Warfarin is metabolized at 1A2. It is because of this complicated metabolism (and because of the protein binding–vitamin K interrelationships and the drug's narrow therapeutic window) that warfarin is so sensitive to inhibition and induction by so many drugs. In the *Physicians' Desk Reference* (2001), the list of warfarin interactions takes up three columns. In general, if a patient is taking warfarin, careful monitoring of anticoagulation (prothrombin time and international normalized ratio) and of levels of drugs coadministered is necessary. Nearly every psychotropic drug has been implicated in a warfarin interaction.

Antiplatelet Drugs

The thienopyridines ticlopidine and clopidogrel are inhibitors of platelet function. These agents reduce the incidence of atherosclerotic events in patients with histories of myocardial infarction, peripheral vascular disease, or stroke. Ticlopidine is a potent, specific inhibitor of 2C19. Donahue et al. (1999) reported on ticlopidine and its effects on phenytoin clearance via 2C19. Clopidogrel is an inhibitor of 2C9. In our search of the literature, we found no reports of in vivo randomized, double-blind pharmacokinetic studies of clopidogrel. In theory, clopidogrel could increase serum concentrations of and hence side-effect profiles of phenytoin, tamoxifen, tolbutamide, warfarin, fluvastatin, zafirlukast, oral hypoglycemics, and many of the nonsteroidal anti-inflammatory drugs (Plavix package insert 1997).

Calcium-Channel Blockers

General Drug Interactions

3A4 inhibition *of* CCBs. All calcium-channel blockers (CCBs) are substrates at 3A4 for oxidative biotransformation. Caution is prudent whenever a CCB is coadministered with potent 3A4 inhibitors, especially erythromycin, clarithromycin, ketoconazole, ritonavir, nefazodone, and grapefruit juice. For example, ketoconazole increased the mean area under the curve (AUC) and maximal drug concentration (C_{max}) of nisoldipine and its active metabolite in a randomized crossover trial in healthy volunteers (Heinig et al. 1999).

The dihydropyridine CCBs became available in the late 1980s, and, by 1991, the first reports of interactions with orally administered drugs of this class and grapefruit juice had appeared. Grapefruit juice causes an increase in the AUC and C_{max} of these drugs. Intravenous administration of CCBs in combination with grapefruit juice has no such effect, and compared with 3A4 inhibition by a potent inhibitor such as erythromycin, grapefruit juice does not prolong the half-lives of CCBs, indication that there is no interaction hepatically and that the interaction may be entirely in the gut wall. The exact compound responsible for this first-pass effect of grapefruit juice has yet to be identified (Bailey et al. 1996, 1998; Fuhr et al. 1998).

3A4 inhibition *by* CCBs. Diltiazem is the most potent 3A4 inhibitor of this class of drugs. There have been case reports of cisapride toxicity with other CCBs as well (Posicor package insert 1997; Thomas et al. 1998). Diltiazem also inhibits tamoxifen. Ocran et al. (1999) described tacrolimus toxicity in a renal transplant recipient being given mibefradil, and CCB inhibition of 3A4 has been exploited to reduce the cost of cyclosporine therapy (see Chapter 15).

2D6 inhibition *by* CCBs. Mibefradil, which is no longer on the United States market, is an example of an agent with potent inhibition at both 2D6 and 3A4. Mibefradil was voluntarily with-

126

■ CALCIUM-CHANNEL BLOCKERS

Drug	Metabolism site(s)	Enzyme(s) inhibited	Enzyme(s) induced
Amlodipine	3A4	None known	None known
Diltiazem	3A4, 2D6	3A4	None known
Felodipine	3A4	None known	None known
Isradipine	None known	None known	None known
Mibefradil[1]	3A4	**3A4**[a], **2D6**[a]	None known
Nifedipine	3A4, ?2D6	None known	None known
Nisoldipine	3A4, 2D6	None known	None known
Verapamil	3A4, 2C9, 2E1	3A4	None known

[1]No longer available, because of adverse drug interactions based on inhibition of 2D6 and 3A4 substrates.

[a]Potent (bold type).
[b]Moderate.
[c]Mild.

drawn in 1998 after multiple reports of life-threatening drug interactions. Mullins et al. (1998) reported one death and three survivors after cardiogenic shock associated with mibefradil administered with dihydropyridine CCBs and β-blockers (2D6).

Induction of CCBs. Rifampin is a potent inducer of many P450 enzymes. Oral rifampin seems to have induced nifedipine metabolism in six healthy volunteers in a randomized, double crossover study, as evidenced by increased oral clearance and decreased bioavailability, with a calculated extraction of nifedipine in gut wall mucosa being significantly increased. Intravenous administration of nifedipine in the same subjects was not associated with altered nifedipine pharmacokinetics (Holtbecker et al. 1996). (See "Antimycobacterials and Antitubercular Agents" in Chapter 12.)

Psychotropic Interactions

Triazolobenzodiazepines. Triazolobenzodiazepines are all inhibited by the 3A4 inhibitors diltiazem and verapamil. In a randomized, three-phase crossover study in healthy volunteers, diltiazem increased the AUC, C_{max}, and half-life of triazolam, which worsened triazolam's sedative effects (Kosuge et al. 1997). Ahonen et al. (1996) randomly assigned 30 patients who were to undergo coronary artery bypass surgery to diltiazem or placebo in addition to standard cardiac anesthesia with midazolam and alfentanil. In this double-blind study, the researchers found that diltiazem increased the mean concentration-time curves of both midazolam and alfentanil and increased the half-lives of the drugs by 43% and 50%, respectively. Extubation of the patients who received diltiazem occurred 2.5 hours later than extubation of the control subjects, a significant difference.

Buspirone. The CCBs verapamil and diltiazem increased the AUC of buspirone in healthy volunteers, diltiazem to a significantly greater degree than verapamil. Buspirone side effects were greater in the patients given diltiazem than in the placebo group (Lamberg et al. 1998).

Fluoxetine. An 80-year-old man developed orthostatic hypotension and weakness after fluoxetine was added to long-standing nifedipine therapy (Azaz-Livshits and Danenberg 1997). There were no serum levels to assist in this evaluation, and we found no other reports that would have explained the inhibition of nifedipine, a substrate of 3A, by the 2D6 inhibitor fluoxetine.

Summary

The CCBs have noxious side effects that may be dose limiting. Inhibition of CCBs by 3A4 inhibitors, including grapefruit juice, leads to orthostasis, hypotension, and tachycardia. Diltiazem and verapamil are inhibitors of 3A4 metabolism and cause increases in side effects of triazolobenzodiazepines, buspirone, alfentanil, and potentially any other 3A4 substrate.

Hydroxymethylglutaryl–Coenzyme A Reductase Inhibitors

Hydroxymethylglutaryl–coenzyme A (HMG-CoA) reductase inhibitors decrease plasma cholesterol levels by inhibiting cholesterol synthesis in the liver. Toxicity may lead to myopathy, muscle toxicity, and rhabdomyolysis (Gruer et al. 1999). Lovastatin, simvastatin, and atorvastatin are 3A4 substrates. When coadministered with potent 3A4 inhibitors, HMG-CoA toxicity may result. Pravastatin is apparently not metabolized at 3A4 and is not affected by the inhibitors itraconazole and grapefruit juice (Neuvonen et al. 1998). Cerivastatin seems to be metabolized at several P450 sites, with 3A4 being the major site in vitro (Boberg et al. 1997). Cerivastatin is effective at low doses, making even modest interactions less dangerous. Pravastatin and cerivastatin seem to be less susceptible to potent inhibition by 3A4 inhibitors because of these characteristics. Although Muck (1998) stated that cerivastatin appears to "lack clinically relevant interactions with digoxin, warfarin, antacid, cimetidine, nifedipine, omeprazole, erythromycin and itraconazole" (p. 15), Muck and colleagues (1999) later reported that cyclosporine resulted in three- to fivefold increases in cerivastatin and its active metabolites in kidney transplant recipients. Kantola et al.

(1999) also found a "modest" interaction between cerivastatin and itraconazole, which led to increases in the C_{max}, AUC, and half-life of cerivastatin in healthy volunteers. The interactions of this latest "statin" are not yet fully studied. Concomitant use of HMG-CoA reductase inhibitors and potent 3A4 inhibitors should be avoided, the dose of HMG-CoA should be reduced, or cerivastatin (less potent but effective) should be used.

■ GASTROINTESTINAL AGENTS

General Drug Interactions

Cisapride

Cisapride, which was prescribed for upper gastrointestinal motility disorders, was removed from the United States market in July 2000. The agent had little effect on the metabolism of other drugs. However, cisapride is extremely cardiotoxic at supratherapeutic doses and, like terfenadine, is a substrate of (metabolized at) 3A4. Inhibitors of 3A4 may cause arrhythmia and torsades de pointes. In a March 2000 Talk Paper, the U.S. Food and Drug Administration (2000) cited 341 cases of cardiac arrhythmia and 80 fatalities from serious interactions with cisapride between 1993 and 1999. Cisapride was contraindicated with the following: macrolides, azole antifungals, protease inhibitors, phenothiazines, class IA and III antiarrhythmics, tricyclic antidepressants, antipsychotic medications, grapefruit juice, some fluoroquinolones, and other substances (Propulcid 2000). Despite "black box" warnings and direct mailings to all physicians, these drugs continued to be coprescribed, leading to withdrawal of cisapride from the market.

H_2-Receptor Blockers

Cimetidine is involved in numerous drug interactions at multiple enzyme sites. Because most of cimetidine's premarketing research was conducted in the early 1980s, microsomal and drug-interaction studies are incomplete and results are sometimes conflicting. Cimetidine has been documented to cause decreased clearance and un-

■ GASTROINTESTINAL AGENTS

Drug	Metabolism site(s)	Enzyme(s) inhibited	Enzyme(s) induced
Prokinetics			
Cisapride[1]	3A4	3A4	None known
H₂-receptor blockers			
Cimetidine	None known	3A4, 2D6, 1A2, 2C9[2]	None known
Famotidine	None known	None known	None known
Nizatidine	None known	None known	None known
Ranitidine	None known	1A2, 2C9, 2C19[b]	None known
Proton pump inhibitors			
Lansoprazole	3A4, 2C19	None known	1A2[c]
Omeprazole	3A4, 2C19	2C19	1A2
Pantoprazole	3A4, 2C19	None known	None known
Rabeprazole	3A4, 2C19	None known	None known

[1]Cardiotoxic pro-drug; removed from the United States market in July 2000.
[2]Minor pathway.

[a]Potent (bold type).
[b]Moderate.
[c]Mild.

wanted side effects of nonsteroidal anti-inflammatory drugs and warfarin (2C9), theophylline and olanzapine (1A2) (Szymanski et al. 1991), propranolol and other β-blockers (2D6), and tricyclics (2D6?). Ranitidine is associated with almost none of these interactions, although there are case reports of interactions between ranitidine and phenytoin (Tse et al. 1993). Perhaps the greatest problem with cimetidine is its availability as an over-the-counter preparation. Physicians must ask patients about use of this drug before prescribing any drug with a narrow therapeutic window or when evaluating a potential adverse event. Famotidine is associated with no reported metabolic interactions (Humphries 1987). H_2-receptor blockers also reduce the plasma concentrations of ketoconazole, indomethacin, and chlorpromazine by altering their absorption. (For a full discussion of many of these interactions, see the review of antiulcer drugs by Negro [1998].)

Proton Pump Inhibitors

Proton pump inhibitors inhibit enzymes on the apical surface of parietal cells in the stomach, preventing secretion of gastric acid. Some of these agents interfere with absorption of drugs such as digoxin and ketoconazole. Omeprazole is the oldest proton pump inhibitor and the drug with potential for pharmacokinetic interactions. 2C19 inhibition occurs with administration of omeprazole, affecting diazepam, warfarin, carbamazepine, and phenytoin metabolism (Petersen 1995). Omeprazole and lansoprazole *induce* 1A2 and may affect theophylline and caffeine. Pantoprazole has none of these effects, a conclusion drawn from a review of the literature and findings of randomized studies involving healthy volunteers (Hartmann et al. 1999; Steinijans et al. 1996). Rabeprazole also seems to be free of metabolic interactions (Lew 1999).

Psychotropic Drug Interactions

H_2-Receptor Blockers

Sanders et al. (1993) conducted a head-to-head study of ranitidine and cimetidine. Midazolam was added to steady-state H_2-receptor blockers in a randomized, double-blind crossover study involving healthy volunteers. These investigators found a significant difference in impairment (pharmacodynamic effect) of 2.5 hours in the cimetidine treatment group compared with the ranitidine treatment group, and the decrement was evident in cognitive and psychomotor functions but was not subjectively reported by the subjects. The "pan-inhibitor" cimetidine worsened side effects of midazolam by inhibiting 3A4.

Proton Pump Inhibitors

Omeprazole is an inhibitor of 2C19. Omeprazole's effect on diazepam levels was studied in poor and rapid metabolizers of omeprazole. In a double-blind crossover study, diazepam was administered intravenously after steady state had been achieved with omeprazole therapy (Andersson et al. 1990). Diazepam metabolism was slowed significantly in the rapid metabolizers (i.e., the rapid metabolizers became phenotypic poor metabolizers) by omeprazole. The poor metabolizers showed no apparent interaction.

■ ORAL HYPOGLYCEMICS

The thiazolidinedione antidiabetic agents have been designed to improve insulin resistance in patients with type II diabetes (diabetes mellitus).

3A4 Induction by Oral Hypoglycemics

Troglitazone has been shown to decrease cyclosporine concentrations in renal transplant recipients (Kaplan et al. 1998). The drug is a known 3A4 inducer; it can decrease the serum concentration of 3A4 substrates, including protease inhibitors and oral contraceptives. In in vitro studies of human liver microsomes, troglitazone is as potent an inducer as rifampicin. Rosiglitazone, in the manufacturer's randomized, open-label, crossover study involving 28 healthy volunteers, produced no clinically significant decrease in nifedipine pharmacokinetics, nifedipine being a probe drug for 3A4 interactions. Both drugs are linked to hepatocellular injury independent of the P450-mediated interactions. In March 2000, the U.S. Food and Drug Administration requested that troglitazone be removed from the United States market, and the manufacturer complied ("Rezulin to Be Withdrawn From the Market" 2000). Troglitazone has greater hepatotoxicity than do other drugs in this class. Pioglitazone is the newest thiazolidiendione for treatment of type II diabetes. This agent is partially metabolized by 3A4, and drug interaction studies have not been conducted. Postmarketing surveillance has revealed that pioglitazone is less hepatotoxic than others in this class.

■ REFERENCES

Abernethy DR, Schwartz JB: Calcium-antagonist drugs. N Engl J Med 341:1447–1457, 1999

Ahonen J, Olkkola KT, Salmenpera M, et al: Effect of diltiazem on midazolam and alfentanil disposition in patients undergoing coronary artery bypass grafting. Anesthesiology 85:1246–1252, 1996

Andersson T, Cederberg C, Edvardsson, et al: Effect of omeprazole treatment on diazepam plasma levels in slow versus normal rapid metabolizers of omeprazole. Clin Pharmacol Ther 47:79–85, 1990

Andrews PA: Interactions with ciprofloxacin and erythromycin leading to aminophylline toxicity. Nephrol Dial Transplant 13:1006–1008, 1998

Azaz-Livshits TL, Danenberg HD: Tachycardia, orthostatic hypotension and profound weakness due to concomitant use of fluoxetine and nifedipine. Pharmacopsychiatry 30:274–275, 1997

Bailey DG, Bend JR, Arnold JM, et al: Erythromycin-felodipine interaction: magnitude, mechanism, and comparison with grapefruit juice. Clin Pharmacol Ther 60:25–33, 1996

Bailey DG, Kreeft JH, Munoz C, et al: Grapefruit juice-felodipine interaction: effect of naringin and 6′,7′-dihydroxybergamottin in humans. Clin Pharmacol Ther 64:248–256, 1998

Batty KT, Davis TM, Ilett KF, et al: The effect of ciprofloxacin on theophylline pharmacokinetics in healthy subjects. Br J Clin Pharmacol 39:305–311, 1995

Benedek IH, Davidson AF, Pieniaszek HJ Jr: Enzyme induction by moricizine: time course and extent in healthy subjects. J Clin Pharmacol 34:167–175, 1994

Boberg M, Angerbauer R, Fey P, et al: Metabolism of cerivastatin by human liver microsomes in vitro: characterization of primary metabolic pathways and of cytochrome P450 isozymes involved. Drug Metab Dispos 25:321–331, 1997

Buchert E, Woosley RL: Clinical implications of variable antiarrhythmic drug metabolism. Pharmacogenetics 2:2–11, 1992

Davies AJ, Harindra V, McEwan A, et al: Cardiotoxic effect with convulsions in terfenadine overdose. BMJ 298:325, 1989

Depre M, Van Hecken A, Verbesselt R, et al: Effect of multiple doses of montelukast, a CysLT1 receptor antagonist, on digoxin pharmacokinetics in healthy volunteers. J Clin Pharmacol 39:941–944, 1999

DeVane CL, Markowitz JS, Hardesty SJ, et al: Fluvoxamine-induced theophylline toxicity. Am J Psychiatry 154:1317–1318, 1997

Donahue S, Flockhart DA, Abernethy DR: Ticlopidine inhibits phenytoin clearance. Clin Pharmacol Ther 66:563–568, 1999

Food and Drug Administration: Janssen Pharmaceutica stops marketing cisapride in the US (Talk Paper T00-14). Rockville, MD, National Press Office, March 23, 2000 [www.fda.gov/bbs/topics/ANSWERS/ANS01007.html]

Fuhr U, Maier-Bruggemann A, Blume H, et al: Grapefruit juice increases oral nimodipine bioavailability. Int J Clin Pharmacol Ther 36:126–132, 1998

Grace AA, Camm AJ: Quinidine. N Engl J Med 338:35–44, 1998

Gruer PJ, Vega JM, Mercuri MF, et al: Concomitant use of cytochrome P450 3A4 inhibitors and simvastatin. Am J Cardiol 84:811–815, 1999

Hartmann M, Zech K, Bliesath H, et al: Pantoprazole lacks induction of CYP1A2 activity in man. Int J Clin Pharmacol Ther 37:159–164, 1999

Heinig R, Adelmann HG, Ahr G: The effect of ketoconazole on the pharmacokinetics, pharmacodynamics and safety of nisoldipine. Eur J Clin Pharmacol 55:57–60, 1999

Holtbecker N, Fromm MF, Kroemer HK, et al: The nifedipine-rifampin interaction: evidence for induction of gut wall metabolism. Drug Metab Dispos 24:1121–1123, 1996

Humphries TJ: Famotidine: a notable lack of drug interactions. Scand J Gastroenterol Suppl 134:55–60, 1987

Kantola T, Kivisto KT, Neuvonen PJ: Effect of itraconazole on cerivastatin pharmacokinetics. Eur J Clin Pharmacol 54:851–855, 1999

Kaplan B, Friedman G, Jacobs M, et al: Potential interaction of troglitazone and cyclosporine. Transplantation 27:1399–1400, 1998

Katial RK, Stelzle RC, Bonner MW, et al: A drug interaction between zafirlukast and theophylline. Arch Intern Med 158:1713–1715, 1998

Kobayashi K, Nakajima M, Chiba K, et al: Inhibitory effects of antiarrhythmic drugs on phenacetin O-deethylation catalysed by human CYP1A2. Br J Clin Pharmacol 45:361–368, 1998

Kosuge K, Nishimoto M, Kimura M, et al: Enhanced effect of triazolam with diltiazem. Br J Clin Pharmacol 43:367–372, 1997

Lamberg TS, Kivisto KT, Neuvonen PJ: Effects of verapamil and diltiazem on the pharmacokinetics and pharmacodynamics of buspirone. Clin Pharmacol Ther 63:640–645, 1998

Lew EA: Review article: pharmacokinetic concerns in the selection of anti-ulcer therapy. Aliment Pharmacol Ther 13 (suppl 5):11–6, 1999

Lilja JJ, Kivisto KT, Neuvonen PJ: Grapefruit juice increases serum concentrations of atorvastatin and has no effect on pravastatin. Clin Pharmacol Ther 66:118–127, 1999

Loi CM, Young M, Randinitis E, et al: Clinical pharmacokinetics of troglitazone. Clin Pharmacokinet 37:91–104, 1999

Monahan BP, Ferguson CL, Killeavy ES, et al: Torsades de pointes occurring in association with terfenadine use. JAMA 264:2788–2790, 1990

Morike KE, Roden DM: Quinidine-enhanced beta-blockade during treatment with propafenone in extensive metabolizer human subjects. Clin Pharmacol Ther 55:28–34, 1994

Muck W: Rational assessment of the interaction profile of cerivastatin supports its low propensity for drug interactions. Drugs 56 (suppl 1):15–23, 1998

Muck W, Mai I, Fritsche L, et al: Increase in cerivastatin systemic exposure after single and multiple dosing in cyclosporine-treated kidney transplant recipients. Clin Pharmacol Ther 65:251–261, 1999

Mullins ME, Horowitz BZ, Linden DH, et al: Life-threatening interaction of mibefradil and beta-blockers with dihydropyridine calcium channel blockers. JAMA 280:157–158, 1998

Negro RD: Pharmacokinetic drug interactions with anti-ulcer drugs. Clin Pharmacokinet 35:135–150, 1998

Neuvonen PJ, Kantola T, Kivisto KT: Simvastatin but not pravastatin is very susceptible to interaction with the CYP3A4 inhibitor itraconazole. Clin Pharmacol Ther 63:332–341, 1998

Ocran KW, Plauth M, Mai I, et al: Tacrolimus toxicity due to drug interaction with mibefradil in a patient after liver transplantation. Z Gastroenterol 37:1025–1028, 1999

Petersen KU: Omeprazole and the cytochrome P450 system (review article). Aliment Pharmacol Ther 9:1–9, 1995

Physicians' Desk Reference, 55th Edition. Montvale, NJ, Medical Economics, 2001

Pieniaszek HJ Jr, Davidson AF, Benedek IH: Effect of moricizine on the pharmacokinetics of single-dose theophylline in healthy subjects. Ther Drug Monit 15:199–203, 1993

Plavix package insert. New York, NY, Sanofi/Bristol-Myers Squibb Co, 1997

Posicor package insert. Nutley, NJ, Roche Pharmaceuticals, 1997

Propulsid drug warning. Titusville, NJ, Janssen Pharmaceutica, January 2000

Rasmussen BB, Maenpaa J, Pelkonen O, et al: Selective serotonin reuptake inhibitors and theophylline metabolism in human liver microsomes: potent inhibition by fluvoxamine. Br J Clin Pharmacol 39:151–159, 1995

Rasmussen BB, Jeppesen U, Gaist D, et al: Griseofulvin and fluvoxamine interactions with the metabolism of theophylline. Ther Drug Monit 19:56–62, 1997

Renwick AG: The metabolism of antihistamines and drug interactions: the role of cytochrome P450 enzymes. Clin Exp Allergy 29 (suppl 3):116–124, 1999[1]

Rezulin to be withdrawn from the market. HHS News, US Department of Health and Human Services, March 21, 2000 [www.fda.gov/bbs/topics/NEWS/NEW00721.html]

Sanders LD, Whitehead C, Gildersleve CD: Interaction of H2-receptor antagonists and benzodiazepine sedation: a double-blind placebo-controlled investigation of the effects of cimetidine and ranitidine on recovery after intravenous midazolam. Anaesthesia 48:286–292, 1993

Shum L, Pieniaszek HJ Jr, Robinson CA: Pharmacokinetic interactions of moricizine and diltiazem in healthy volunteers. J Clin Pharmacol 36:1161–1168, 1996

Slater JW, Zechnich AD, Haxby DG: Second generation antihistamines: a comparative review. Drugs 57:31–47, 1999

Spinler SA, Gammaitoni A, Charland SL, et al: Propafenone-theophylline interaction. Pharmacotherapy 13:68–71, 1993

---

[1] This entire supplement of *Clinical Experimental Allergy* is devoted to antihistamines, with many articles relevant to this topic for psychiatrists.

Steinijans VW, Huber R, Hartmann M, et al: Lack of pantoprazole drug interactions in man: an updated review. Int J Clin Pharmacol Ther 34: 243–262, 1996

Szymanski S, Lieberman JA, Picou D, et al: A case report of cimetidine-induced clozapine toxicity. J Clin Psychiatry 52:21–22, 1991

Thomas AR, Chan LN, Bauman JL, et al: Prolongation of the QT interval related to cisapride-diltiazem interaction. Pharmacotherapy 18:381–385, 1998

Tse CS, Akinwande KI, Biallowons K: Phenytoin concentration elevation subsequent to ranitidine administration. Ann Pharmacother 27:1448–1451, 1993

Upton RA: Pharmacokinetic interactions between theophylline and other medication (part I). Clin Pharmacokinet 20:66–80, 1991

Van Hecken A, Depre M, Verbesselt R, et al: Effect of montelukast on the pharmacokinetics and pharmacodynamics of warfarin in healthy volunteers. J Clin Pharmacol 39:495–500, 1999

Wei X, Dai R, Zhai S, et al: Inhibition of human liver cytochrome P450 1A2 by the class 1B antiarrhythmics mexiletine, lidocaine, and tocainide. J Pharmacol Exp Ther 289:853–858, 1999

Woosley RL: Cardiac actions of antihistamines. Annu Rev Pharmacol Toxicol 36:233–252, 1996

Yap TG, Camm AJ: The current cardiac safety situation with antihistamines. Clin Exp Allergy 29 (suppl 1):15–24, 1999

Zevin S, Benowitz NL: Drug interactions with tobacco smoking: an update. Clin Pharmacokinet 36:425–438, 1999

12

INFECTIOUS DISEASES

Antimicrobials are the second most commonly prescribed class of medications in the United States. These drugs are associated with many P450-mediated interactions. Antimalarials and antiparasitic drugs are not covered in this book, because they are not regularly encountered in general medical practice. The antimicrobials with significant P450 activity, as both inducers and inhibitors of enzymes, include macrolide, fluoroquinolone, and streptogramin antibiotics; imidazole antifungals; antimycobacterials; and antiretrovirals. Each of these P450-active antimicrobial classes is dealt with in a separate section below.

> Reminder: In this chapter, only P450-mediated interactions are discussed. Interactions due to displaced protein-binding, alterations in absorption or excretion, and pharmacodynamic interactions are not covered.

■ ANTIBIOTICS

Macrolides

General Drug Interactions

Macrolide antibiotics are known for inhibiting the metabolism of drugs dependent on 3A4 for metabolism—erythromycin and clarithromycin being the most potent.

Cyclosporine. A case has been reported of severe cyclosporine toxicity in a transplant recipient who was concomitantly given clarithromycin (Biaxin) (Spicer et al. 1997). (See Chapter 15.)

■ MACROLIDES

Drug	Metabolism site(s)	Enzyme(s) inhibited	Enzyme(s) induced
Azithromycin	3A4	3A4[c]	None known
Clarithromycin	3A4	**3A4**[a]	None known
Dirithromycin	3A4	None known	None known
Erythromycin	3A4	**3A4**[a]	None known
Rokitamycin	3A4	3A4[b,c]	None known

[a]Potent (bold type).
[b]Moderate.
[c]Mild to not inhibited.

Rifamycin.   Clarithromycin can increase serum levels of rifamycin (rifampin), causing neutropenia and uveitis (Griffith et al. 1995).

Sildenafil.   Sildenafil's (Viagra) package insert (2000) states that erythromycin increases sildenafil's area under the curve (AUC) by 182%. The clinical significance of this increase is unknown.

Calcium-channel blockers.   Calcium-channel blockers are inhibited by macrolides (see "Cardiovascular Agents" in Chapter 11), and this inhibition increases the risk of orthostasis and falls.

Hydroxymethylglutaryl–coenzyme A reductase inhibitors.   Erythromycin increases the AUC and maximal drug concentration (C_{max}) of simvastatin, a hydroxymethylglutaryl–coenzyme A (HMG-CoA) reductase inhibitor, as evidenced by a randomized, double-blind study involving healthy volunteers. This finding is concerning, because toxicity of these agents may lead to rhabdomyolysis (Kantola et al. 1998). (See Chapter 11.)

Psychotropic Interactions

Pimozide.   There have been two reports of sudden death with coadministration of pimozide, an antipsychotic approved for use in patients with Tourette's syndrome (motor and vocal tics), and clarithromycin. Pimozide prolongs QT intervals; therefore, electrocardiographic monitoring is required with pimozide use. Pimozide is a potent inhibitor of 2D6 and a moderate inhibitor of 3A4. The drug is metabolized mainly at 3A4, with some 1A2 contribution (Desta et al. 1998, 1999). We recommend that pimozide not be used with any macrolide antibiotics, and patients must be warned about other moderate to potent 3A4 inhibitors, including grapefruit juice.

Triazolobenzodiazepines.   Prospective, double-blind clinical studies involving small numbers of healthy volunteers have revealed that erythromycin increases the AUC, decreases oral clearance, and prolongs the elimination half-lives of midazolam and alprazolam (Luurila et al. 1996; Yasui et al. 1996). Most of these formal studies did not reveal significant adverse or prolonged pharmacodynamic effects (oversedation or decreased motor performance), although saccadic eye movements were significantly altered from 15 minutes to 6 hours in one early study by Olkkola et al. (1993). In one controlled, double-blind study, women exhibited a greater extent of interaction with clarithromycin and midazolam than did men (Gorski et al. 1998).

Case reports suggest that some patients may be at risk for prolonged or exaggerated effects when these drugs are combined. Delirium was reported when a patient taking triazolam was given erythromycin (Tokinaga et al. 1996). A healthy male who had been taking flunitrazepam and fluoxetine regularly for depression and sleep apnea developed delirium when clarithromycin was added to his regimen for a respiratory infection (Pollak et al. 1995). The authors of the report thought that the delirium was due to fluoxetine intoxication (which rarely causes delirium), but we believe that the clarithromycin probably increased the effects of the benzodiazepine, which is partially metabolized at 3A4. A child experienced prolonged unconsciousness after minor surgery when administered midazolam while taking prophylactic erythromycin (Hiller et al. 1990). Benzodiazepines that are glucuronidated (and therefore not dependent on phase I metabolism), such as lorazepam, oxazepam and temazepam, are without these problems. Azithromycin and dirithromycin mildy inhibit 3A4 and are also without these interactions, as demonstrated in clinical trials and as evidenced by the lack of clinical reports of difficulties (Rapp 1998; Watkins et al. 1997). Rokitamycin needs further clinical study; in vitro human liver enzyme studies indicate that this agent may inhibit 3A4-catalyzed triazolam α-hydroxylation (Zhao et al. 1999).

Buspirone. In a randomized, double-blind study involving healthy volunteers, Kivisto et al. (1997) found that erythromycin increases the AUC of buspirone sixfold, causing psychomotor impairment and an increase in reported buspirone side effects.

Carbamazepine. Carbamazepine toxicity with concomitant use of erythromycin was first reported by Carranco et al. in 1985. Carbamazepine is metabolized at 3A4, which may be inhibited by macrolides and other 3A4 inhibitors (Spina et al. 1996).

Summary

The macrolide antibiotics clarithromycin and erythromycin, and potentially the newer macrolide rokitamycin, are potent inhibitors of 3A4 and have been shown to increase unwanted side effects of medications that are dependent on this enzyme for metabolism. Clarithromycin and erythromycin should not be administered with any medication that both requires metabolism at 3A4 and has known cardiac or other life-threatening effects (i.e., a narrow therapeutic window).

Fluoroquinolones

Fluoroquinolone antibiotics are known for being inhibitors of 1A2, with ciprofloxacin and enoxacin being the most potent inhibitors.

General Drug Interactions

   Xanthines.   Fluoroquinolones affect the metabolism of the xanthine derivatives theophylline, caffeine, and, to some extent, theobromine. These compounds are among the most widely consumed compounds in beverages and pharmaceutical preparations (Robson 1992). Decreased theophylline and caffeine clearance with administration of quinolone antibiotics has been reported since the 1980s (Mizuki et al. 1996). Kinzig-Schippers et al. (1998, 1999) investigated the pharmacokinetics of rufloxacin, pefloxacin, and enoxacin in randomized crossover studies involving healthy volunteers. These researchers found that enoxacin and pefloxacin decrease caffeine clearance. In a separate study, however, theophylline pharmacokinetics were not altered by rufloxacin.

   Warfarin.   The U.S. Food and Drug Administration reported enhanced warfarin anticoagulation with norfloxacin coadministration, but controlled studies found no such effect. The prothrombin time and international normalized ratio of warfarin should be monitored when these antibiotics are coadministered. The enhanced anticoagulation may not be merely a P450-mediated effect.

   Smoking.   Grepafloxacin (a fluoroquinolone that independently prolongs QTc and has been removed from the U.S. market)

■ FLUOROQUINOLONES

Drug	Metabolism	Enzyme(s) inhibited	Enzyme(s) induced
Ciprofloxacin	?	**1A2**,[a] 3A4	None known
Enoxacin	?	**1A2**[a]	None known
Gatifloxacin	Renal excretion/?	None known	None known
Grepafloxacin[1]	1A2, 3A4	1A2	1A2[b]
Levofloxacin	Renal excretion	None known	None known
Moxifloxacin	Not P450	None known	None known
Norfloxacin	Renal excretion/?	1A2, 3A4	None known
Ofloxacin	Renal excretion	1A2[c]	None known
Rufloxacin	?	None known	None known
Sparfloxacin[1]	Phase II	1A2, 3A4[c]	None known
Trovafloxacin	Phase II	None known	None known

Note. ? = Unknown.
[1]Prolongs the QTc interval and removed from the United States market.

[a]Potent (bold type).
[c]Moderate.
[d]Mild.

clearance has been found to be increased in smokers by 35%–43%. Clinical efficacy did not seem to be affected in initial premarketing clinical trials. Chronic cigarette smoking induces metabolism at 1A2, increasing clearance of drugs dependent on this enzyme for metabolism (Glaxo Wellcome Inc. package insert 1999).

Psychotropic Interactions

Tricyclic antidepressants. The *N*-demethylation of amitriptyline and imipramine occurs at 1A2, as does the partial metabolism of other tricyclics (clomipramine and cyclobenzaprine). Despite this knowledge, there are no reports of adverse interactions between tricyclic compounds and fluoroquinolones.

Clozapine. In a case report, Markowitz et al. (1997) suggested that adding ciprofloxacin to the regimen of a patient taking clozapine increased the clozapine levels by 80%.

Diazepam. In a controlled, double-blind study in which 12 healthy volunteers were administered ciprofloxacin for 7 days, serum concentrations of diazepam were increased after a single dose of ciprofloxacin (Kamali et al. 1993). This effect is most likely due to the inhibition of 3A4-metabolized diazepam by ciprofloxacin, because diazepam has not been shown to be metabolized by 1A2.

Tacrine. The hydroxylation of tacrine occurs at 1A2. In an open, randomized crossover study involving 18 healthy volunteers, fluvoxamine was a very potent inhibitor of tacrine metabolism (Larsen et al. 1999). This level of inhibition might enhance tacrine hepatotoxicity. Studies of coadministration of fluoroquinolones and tacrine have not been published to date, but we recommend that this combination not be given until further data are available.

Summary

Quinolones are inhibitors of 1A2. Therefore, when quinolones are administered with drugs that require metabolism at this enzyme, the latter agents are at risk of being inhibited and reaching toxic levels. Drugs with significant adverse reactions or toxicity that are metabolized at 1A2 include warfarin, theophylline, tacrine, and caffeine. There are reports of clozapine toxicity and increased serum diazepam concentrations with fluoroquinolone coadministration. We also caution against the use of these antibiotics with tricyclic antibiotics and tacrine. (See Chapter 6 for further discussion.)

Streptogramins

Quinupristin/dalfopristin is a new combination antibiotic administered intravenously and used to treat resistant infections caused by gram-positive organisms. Vancomycin was the mainstay for treatment of these resistant infections but is now ineffective in a growing number of patients. This combination drug has been used in a Food and Drug Administration–sanctioned emergency capacity in the United States and is scheduled for general release soon. Quinupristin/dalfopristin is a potent inhibitor of 3A4. In in vivo studies involving healthy volunteers, dalfopristin/quinupristin increased the serum levels of cyclosporine, midazolam, and nifedipine ("Quinupristin/Dalfopristin" 1999).

■ ANTIFUNGALS: AZOLES AND TERBINAFINE

Azoles

General Drug Interactions: Inhibition by Azoles

Azole antifungals are known to be inhibitors of 3A4; ketoconazole is often used as a "probe" drug to determine indirectly whether a new drug is metabolized at 3A4. Fluconazole inhibits 3A4 mildly but is a potent inhibitor of 2C9.

HMG-CoA reductase inhibitors.   Azoles affect the pharmacokinetics of simvastatin and lovastatin (HMG-CoA reductase inhibitors used to decrease low-density lipoprotein levels in hypercholesterolemia). Small doses of itraconazole greatly increase plasma concentrations of lovastatin and simvastatin but not fluvastatin. These increased serum levels of HMG-CoA reductase inhibitors

■ ANTIFUNGALS

Drug	Metabolism site(s)	Enzyme(s) inhibited	Enzyme(s) induced
Azoles			
Fluconazole	?	**2C9**,[a] 3A4[b]	None known
Itraconazole	3A4	**3A4**[a]	None known
Ketoconazole	3A4	**3A4**[a]	None known
Miconazole	3A4	None or mildly inhibited	None known
Other antifungals			
Terbinafine	?	2D6	None known

Note. ? = Unknown.
[a]Potent (bold type).
[b]Moderate.
[c]Mild.

can lead to skeletal muscle toxicity (Kivisto et al. 1998; Neuvonen et al. 1998). In the intraconazole manufacturer's package insert (Sporanox package insert 2000), it was reported that rhabdomyolysis occurred in renal transplant recipients given cyclosporine, itraconazole, and HMG-CoA reductase inhibitors. (See "Hydroxymethylglutaryl–Coenzyme A Reductase Inhibitors" in Chapter 11 for further discussion.)

Cyclosporine.   Interactions between HMG-CoA reductase inhibitors and itraconazole and cyclosporine are discussed in the previous paragraph. Ketoconazole inhibition has been used in an attempt to reduce the amount spent on cyclosporine in transplant recipients, with mixed results. (See "Immunosuppressants" in Chapter 15.)

Fluconazole.   Fluconazole is the azole antifungal with the safest profile in terms of 3A4 drug interactions and is the systemic antifungal of choice in human immunodeficiency virus (HIV)–positive patients who are taking 3A4 inhibitors such as ritonavir. However, fluconazole is a potent inhibitor of 2C9, the enzyme responsible for the metabolism of phenytoin (the *S*-enantiomer [more active enantiomer] of warfarin) and oral hypoglycemics. Fluconazole has increased phenytoin levels and prothrombin times in healthy volunteers. Fluconazole may also inhibit the metabolism of nonsteroidal anti-inflammatory drugs, potentially worsening gastrointestinal side effects.

General Drug Interactions: Induction of Azoles

Azoles can be induced at 3A4 (i.e., their plasma concentrations can be reduced) by carbamazepine, phenobarbital, phenytoin, and rifampin, reducing their antifungal efficacy.

Psychotropic Interactions

Buspirone.   In a double-blind, randomized, crossover study, healthy volunteers received buspirone and either itraconazole or erythromycin (Kivisto et al. 1997). Psychomotor tests were administered and plasma concentrations, half-lives, and AUCs were determined. Subjects had increased serum buspirone concentrations and significant psychomotor impairments and buspirone-related side effects.

Triazolobenzodiazepines.　Triazolobenzodiazepines require metabolism at 3A4 and therefore may be inhibited by the azoles, resulting in increased drowsiness or sedation and increases in other effects of these medications (Backman et al. 1998).

Cortisol.　Sovner and Fogelman (1996) reported that ketoconazole may be effective in patients with treatment-resistant atypical depression. The authors hypothesized that the potent 3A4 inhibitor ketoconazole inhibited the metabolism of endogenous cortisol at this site, assisting in the treatment of atypical depression.

Terbinafine

Terbinafine is a topical and systemic antifungal used to treat dermatophytoses. Abdel-Rahman et al. (1999) recently reported that healthy extensive-metabolizer phenotype volunteers were "converted" to poor metabolizers of dextromethorphan by terbinafine, in vivo evidence that this drug may inhibit 2D6. Concomitant use with other drugs dependent on 2D6 for metabolism (β-blockers, tricyclic antidepressants, codeine) may increase the risk of toxicity of these drugs. Further study is needed.

Summary

The azole antifungal's mechanism of effect is to inhibit P450 fungal enzyme systems. In humans, the antifungals ketoconazole and itraconazole are potent inhibitors of 3A4 and may increase plasma concentrations of cyclosporine, triazolobenzodiazepines, warfarin, vinca alkaloids (antineoplastic agents), felodipine, methylprednisolone, glyburide, phenytoin, rifabutin, ritonavir, saquinavir, nevirapine, tacrolimus, digoxin, some HMG-CoA reductase inhibitors, and any other drugs dependent on 3A4 for metabolism (Albengres et al. 1998). Fluconazole is the only systemic azole antifungal with mild to moderate inhibition at 3A4 and is thus clinically less problematic at this enzyme. Fluconazole is a potent inhibitor at 2C9 and may increase the risk of toxicity of phenytoin, warfarin, nonsteroidal anti-inflammatory drugs, and oral hypoglycemics.

■ ANTIMYCOBACTERIALS/ ANTITUBERCULAR AGENTS

Rifamycins and Isoniazid

General Drug Interactions

P450 induction. Rifampin (rifampicin) and rifabutin were discovered in 1957 and by 1965 were in wide use for the treatment of tuberculosis. It was quickly learned that the agents *decreased* serum levels of many medications. Where the rifamycins are metabolized has not yet been fully determined, but hepatic and gut wall 3A4 is involved. These drugs are now used in combination therapy for *Mycobacterium avium* complex infection, HIV-related tuberculosis, and community-acquired tuberculosis. Rifapentin decreased the C_{max} and AUC of indinavir by 55% and 70%, respectively, placing HIV-positive patients at risk for viral resistance (Temple and Nahata 1999).

The rifamycins induce many P450 enzymes and also induce phase II glucuronidation, specifically the UGT enzyme system (Gallicano et al. 1999).

Reminder: Induction usually takes a few days and may not wear off for several weeks after discontinuation of the inducing drug. Induction of drugs may lead to ineffectiveness and increase morbidity and mortality.

P450 inhibition. Rifamycins can be inhibited (their plasma concentrations can be increased) by drugs that inhibit 3A4, especially clarithromycin, ketoconazole, and the potent protease inhibitors ritonavir and indinavir, leading to toxic rifampin, rifabutin, or rifapentine levels. It is recommended that rifamycin doses be decreased (which may also reduce induction by these medications) when these drugs are administered with potent inhibitors of 3A4 (Strayhorn et al. 1997).

■ ANTIMYCOBACTERIALS

Drug	Metabolism site(s)	Enzyme(s) inhibited	Enzyme(s) induced
Isoniazid	?	2C9, 2E1	2E1
Rifabutin	3A4	None known	3A4, 1A2, 2C9, 2C19[1]
Rifampin	3A4	None known	3A4, 1A2, 2C9, 2C19[1]
Rifapentine	3A4/?	None known	3A4, 2C9

Note. ? = Unknown.
[1]Rifampin and rifabutin induce all enzymes in humans except 2D6 (an enzyme seemingly not induced by anything) and 2E1.

152

Psychotropic Interactions

Zolpidem. Zolpidem is metabolized by 3A4. In a randomized, double-blind, crossover study, the AUC of zolpidem decreased to 27% of the normal range, the peak plasma concentration decreased by 58%, and the clinical effect of zolpidem was reduced when administered with rifampin (Villikka et al. 1997). Similar effects should be found with triazolobenzodiazepines.

Codeine. The concomitant use of rifamycins and codeine or methadone can lead to opiate withdrawal syndromes (Caraco et al. 1997; Holmes 1990; Kreek et al. 1976). (See "Analgesics" in Chapter 15.)

Buspirone. In a placebo-controlled, double-blind study involving healthy volunteers, rifampicin reduced the AUC and C_{max} of buspirone by 91% and 85%, respectively (Kivisto et al. 1999).

Isoniazid. Isoniazid is an old drug (it was developed in the 1950s), and its mechanism of action is still poorly understood. Slow and fast acetylators were first described in reference to this drug. The half-life of isoniazid is influenced by genetic differences in acetyltransferase activity; isoniazid's elimination half-life in rapid acetylators is 50% that in slow acetylators (Douglas and McLeod 1999). Isoniazid has also been found to inhibit the metabolism of phenytoin, implicating isoniazid as an inhibitor of 2C9 (Kay et al. 1985). Isoniazid may have a biphasic effect at 2E1, greatly affecting acetaminophen metabolism. When first administered with acetaminophen, isoniazid acts as an inhibitor and decreases metabolism to the toxic metabolite *N*-acetyl-*p*-benzoquinone. After 2 weeks, isoniazid becomes an inducer and may increase production of acetaminophen's toxic metabolite and cause hepatotoxicity (Chien et al. 1997; Self et al. 1999).

Summary

In general, the antitubercular drugs rifampin, rifabutin, and rifapentine induce metabolism at most P450 enzymes and can significantly decrease the efficacy of drugs dependent on active parent drug for effect. In the case of drugs that are metabolized to toxic metabolites, induction may lead to more rapid or severe toxicity. Isoniazid is a peculiar drug, with many food and drug interactions, and careful monitoring is needed when isoniazid is administered with drugs metabolized at 2C9 and 2E1.

■ ANTIRETROVIRALS

HIV-positive patients are frequently administered multiple drugs (typically, the lower the CD4 count, the more medications a patient takes). Polypharmacy places this group at great risk for drug-drug interactions. Preston et al. (1998) conducted a retrospective review of 165 records in a tertiary care medicine clinic and found 111 potential drug interactions in 82 patients, the interactions most commonly involving clarithromycin, rifabutin, and the tricyclic antidepressants.

The antiretrovirals with P450 considerations are the protease inhibitors and the *non*-nucleoside reverse transcriptase inhibitors (NNRTIs) (see Antiretrovirals table).

The nucleoside reverse transcriptase inhibitors (NRTIs) nucleoside analogues—which include abacavir, didanosine, lamivudine, stavudine, zalcitabine, and zidovudine—and the new acyclic phosphonate analogues of deoxynucleoside monophosphates, cidofovir and adefovir—are excreted predominantly by the kidneys and have short half-lives, making P450-mediated drug interactions unlikely. The NRTIs are subject to induction and inhibition of phase II metabolism.

General Drug Interactions

3A4 Inhibition

Ritonavir is the most potent inhibitor in the protease inhibitor group, and in vitro studies have found its inhibitory potency to be slightly less than that of ketoconazole (von Moltke et al. 1998). The same warnings apply to the protease inhibitors as to ketoconazole, erythromycin, and clarithromycin. These drugs all potently inhibit

154

■ ANTIRETROVIRALS

Drug	Metabolism site(s)	Enzyme(s) inhibited	Enzyme(s) induced
Protease inhibitors			
Amprenavir	3A4	3A4[b]	None known
Indinavir	3A4	**3A4**[a]	None known
Lopinavir/ritonavir	3A4	3A4,[b] 2D6[2]	Glucuronidation (phase II)
Nelfinavir	3A4	3A4,[c] 1A2	None known
Ritonavir[1]	3A4	**3A4**,[a] **2D6**,[a] 2C9,[a] 2C19[a]	3A4[a]
Saquinavir	3A4	3A4[c]	None known
Nonnucleoside reverse transcriptase inhibitors			
Delavirdine	3A4, 2D6	3A4,[b] 2C9, 2C19[2]	None known
Efavirenz	3A4	**3A4**,[a] ?2C9	3A4
Nevirapine	3A4, ?others	None known	3A3, 3A4,[b] 2B6[b,c]

[1]Ritonavir is a potent inhibitor of all enzymes except 1A2, 2B6, and 2E1.
[2]Inhibited in vitro.

[a]Potent (bold type).
[b]Moderate.
[c]Mild.

3A4 and can greatly affect drugs with narrow therapeutic indices. In a patient taking ritonavir for HIV infection, ergotism was a severe complication when a drug that included ergotamine tartrate, belladonna, and phenobarbital was added, because of gastric discomfort, to a regimen that also included fluvoxamine (Liaudet et al. 1999). After 5 days of polypharmacy, with all drugs given at recommended doses, the woman developed pain in both legs, leading to bilateral gangrene of the toes and eventual amputation. Ergots are metabolized at 3A4, which is inhibited by ritonavir and fluvoxamine. (See Chapter 13.)

NNRTIs also inhibit P450 enzymes (see Antiretrovirals table). Efavirenz is a potent inhibitor of 3A4 and, interestingly, also *induces* 3A4 (Sustiva package insert 1999).

The metabolism of antiretrovirals can be inhibited as well, leading to greater serum concentrations of drug, as well as potentially intensifying noxious side effects such as nausea, vomiting, and diarrhea. Cimetidine and clarithromycin have increased nevirapine levels, and ketoconazole increased concentrations of delavirdine (Tseng and Foisy 1997). Some centers have reported using inhibition to advantage: plasma levels (and, theoretically, effectiveness) of saquinavir have been increased clinically with the addition of ritonavir, ketoconazole, or grapefruit juice (but concentrations of the latter are inconsistent).

3A4 Induction

Nevirapine is a 3A4 inducer (Viramune package insert 1996). The drug has been found to reduce the plasma AUC of nelfinavir. In recent postmarketing surveillance, nevirapine was found to induce methadone metabolism, causing methadone withdrawal in some patients and thus necessitating an increase in methadone (Altice et al. 1999). Efavirenz, as noted above, is a potent 3A4 inhibitor, but it also induces 3A4 (Sustiva package insert 1999). Concomitant use with 3A4 metabolites with narrow therapeutic windows warrants caution. Drugs such as tricyclic antidepressants or triazolobenzodiazepines, when taken with efavirenz, will immediately require a lower dose of the psychotropic. This effect is due to efavirenz's inhibition of 3A4. Monitoring of serum levels, side effects, and effectiveness must continue for 2–4 weeks. *Induction* may lead to *decreased* levels of the 3A4-dependent medications, requiring *increased* dosages of them at a later date.

Protease inhibitors are metabolized at 3A4 and can also be induced by the usual potent inducers: phenytoin, carbamazepine, alcohol, rifamycins, and barbiturates. Rifampin and rifapentine induce protease inhibitors and NNRTIs and can decrease serum concentrations, and these actions may lead to viral resistance (decreased sensitivity to the protease inhibitor or nonnucleoside reverse transcriptase inhibitor). St. John's wort was recently found to induce 3A4, decreasing mean plasma indinavir concentrations by 57% and trough levels by 81% (Piscitelli et al. 2000b).

The newest protease inhibitor is a combination drug containing ritonavir and lopinavir. Ritonavir, one of the most potent 3A4 inhibitors, may increase any other coadministered drugs dependent on 3A4 for metabolism (see 3A4 tables in Chapter 5). Interestingly, lopinavir induces glucuronidation. This phase II metabolism induction can greatly reduce levels of the NRTIs zidovudine and abacavir, reducing effectiveness and resulting in viral resistance. Lopinavir has also been found to increase clearance of methadone and ethinyl estradiol (EE). In vitro, lopinavir/ritonavir also inhibits 2D6, but clinical studies are pending (personal communication from C. Koch, Pharm.D., Medical Information Specialist, and R. Hodd, M.D., Medical Director, Abbott Laboratories, December 19, 2000; Kaletra package insert 2000).

Ritonavir, although a potent inhibitor of 3A4, *induces* 3A4 metabolism after a few weeks. Ritonavir has been found to increase the metabolism of meperidine, resulting in increased levels of the neurotoxic metabolite normeperidine, and has been found to reduce the AUC and C_{max} of ethinyl estradiol (EE) (Ouellet et al. 1998; Piscitelli et al. 2000a). There are no reports to date of ritonavir compromising the effectiveness of coadministered protease inhibitors that rely on 3A4 metabolism, and, in fact, ritonavir has recently been introduced as a combination protease inhibitor with lopinavir, as noted above. Ritonavir's induction of the 3A4 enzyme requires further clinical study, and there are no reports of ritonavir being a "pan-inducer." In short, ritonavir has been found to be a "pan-*inhibitor*" of P450 enzymes and a specific *inducer* at 3A4, and lopinavir is an inducer of phase II metabolism, effecting glucuronidation.

Psychotropic Interactions

Triazolobenzodiazepines

A 32-year-old man with HIV infection tolerated midazolam for bronchoscopy while taking zidovudine and lamivudine. Saquinavir was added without problems. However, when he needed another bronchoscopy, the same dose of midazolam necessitated the addition of flumazenil for prolonged sedation, and the patient remained impaired for more than 5 hours (Merry et al. 1997). Midazolam's metabolism was inhibited by the protease inhibitor, prolonging midazolam's sedating effects.

Tricyclic Antidepressants

Tricyclic antidepressants may be affected by ritonavir, because all metabolic routes may be inhibited, leading to toxicity.

Antipsychotics

Clozapine metabolism may be inhibited by ritonavir. For treatment of psychosis in a patient who must take ritonavir, olanzapine may be the best choice, because this drug is metabolized by several enzymes and by phase II.

Methadone and Buprenorphine

In vitro studies involving human microsomes revealed that protease inhibitors inhibit methadone *N*-demethylation and buprenorphine *N*-dealkylation, which could lead to respiratory compromise secondary to opiate toxicity (Iribarne et al. 1998).

Summary

Ritonavir is a very potent "pan-inhibitor," with activity at most P450 enzymes. Whenever a patient is administered ritonavir, caution must be taken with all added drugs that have narrow therapeutic windows. All protease inhibitors are metabolized at 3A4, and all exhibit some inhibition at 3A4. The nonnucleoside reverse transcriptase inhibitor efavirenz is a potent inhibitor of 3A4, and nevirapine, ritonavir, and efavirenz are inducers of 3A4. Lopinavir/ritonavir carries all of the warnings for ritonavir and may also induce the metabolism of methadone, oral contraceptives, and NRTIs via induction of glucuronidation. Metabolism of all protease inhibitors and NNRTIs may be induced by antitubercular drugs like rifampin, leading to ineffectiveness and viral resistance.

■ REFERENCES

Abdel-Rahman SM, Gotschall RR, Kauffman RE, et al: Investigation of terbinafine as a CYP2D6 inhibitor in vivo. Clin Pharmacol Ther 65:465–472, 1999

Albengres E, LeLouet H, Tillement JP: Systemic antifungal agents: drug interactions of clinical significance. Drug Saf 18:83–97, 1998

Altice FL, Friedland GH, Cooney EL: Nevirapine induced opiate withdrawal among injection drug users with HIV infection receiving methadone. AIDS 13:957–962, 1999

Backman JT, Kivisto KT, Olkkola KT, et al: The area under the plasma concentration-time curve for oral midazolam is 400-fold larger during treatment with itraconazole than with rifampicin. Eur J Clin Pharmacol 54:53–58, 1998

Balfour JA, Wiseman LR: Moxifloxacin. Drugs 57:363–373, 1999

Caraco Y, Sheller J, Wood AJ: Pharmacogenetic determinants of codeine induction by rifampin: the impact on codeine's respiratory, psychomotor and miotic effects. J Pharmacol Exp Ther 281:330–336, 1997

Carranco E, Kareus J, Co S, et al: Carbamazepine toxicity induced by concurrent erythromycin therapy. Arch Neurol 42:187–188, 1985

Chien JY, Peter RM, Nolan CM, et al: Influence of polymorphic *N*-acetyltransferase phenotype on the inhibition and induction of acetaminophen bioactivation with long-term isoniazid. Clin Pharmacol Ther 61:24–34, 1997

Desta Z, Kerbusch T, Soukhova N, et al: Identification and characterization of human cytochrome P450 isoforms interacting with pimozide. J Pharmacol Exp Ther 285:428–437, 1998

Desta Z, Kerbusch T, Flockart DA: Effect of clarithromycin on the pharma-cokinetics and pharmacodynamics of pimozide in healthy poor and extensive metabolizers of cytochrome P450 2D6 (CYP2D6). Clin Pharmacol Ther 65:10–20, 1999

Douglas JG, McLeod M: Pharmacokinetic factors in modern drug treatment of tuberculosis. Clin Pharmacokinet 37:127–146, 1999

Eagling VA, Back DJ, Barry MG: Differential inhibition of cytochrome P450 isoforms by the protease inhibitors, ritonavir, saquinavir and indin-avir. Br J Clin Pharmacol 44:190–194, 1997

Efthymiopoulos C: Pharmacokinetics of grepafloxacin. J Antimicrob Chemother 40 (suppl A):35–43, 1997

Gallicano KD, Sahai J, Shukla VK, et al: Induction of zidovudine glucur-onidation and amination pathways by rifampicin in HIV-infected pa-tients. Br J Clin Pharmacol 48:168–179, 1999

Gorski JC, Jones DR, Haehner-Daniels BD, et al: The contribution of intes-tinal and hepatic CYP3A to the interaction between midazolam and clarithromycin. Clin Pharmacol Ther 64:133–143, 1998

Griffith DE, Brown BA, Girard WM, et al: Adverse events associated with high-dose rifabutin in macrolide-containing regimens for the treatment of *Mycobacterium avium* complex lung disease. Clin Infect Dis 21:594–598, 1995

Hiller A, Olkkola KT, Isohanni P, et al: Unconsciousness associated with midazolam and erythromycin. Br J Anaesth 65:826–828, 1990

Holmes VF: Rifampin-induced methadone withdrawal in AIDS (letter). J Clin Psychopharmacol 10:443–444, 1990

Iatsimirskaia E, Tulebaev S, Storozhuk E, et al: Metabolism of rifabutin in human enterocyte and liver microsomes: kinetic parameters, identifica-tion of enzyme systems, and drug interactions with macrolides and an-tifungal agents. Clin Pharmacol Ther 61:554–562, 1997

Iribarne C, Berthou F, Carlhant D, et al: Inhibition of methadone and bu-prenorphine N-dealkylations by three HIV-1 protease inhibitors. Drug Metab Dispos 26:257–260, 1998

Kaletra package insert. Abbott Park, IL, Abbott Laboratories, 2000

Kamali F, Thomas SHL, Edwards C: The influence of steady-state cipro-floxacin on the pharmacokinetics and pharmacodynamics of a single dose of diazepam in healthy volunteers. Eur J Clin Pharmacol 44:365–367, 1993

Kantola T, Kivisto KT, Neuvonen PJ: Erythromycin and verapamil consid-erably increase serum simvastatin and simvastatin acid concentrations. Clin Pharmacol Ther 64:177–182, 1998

160

Kay L, Kampmann JP, Svendsen T, et al: Influence of rifampicin and isoniazid on the kinetics of phenytoin. Br J Clin Pharmacol 20:323–326, 1985

Kinzig-Schippers M, Fuhr U, Cesana M, et al: Absence of effect of rufloxacin on theophylline pharmacokinetics in steady state. Antimicrob Agents Chemother 42:2359–2364, 1998

Kinzig-Schippers M, Fuhr U, Zaigler M, et al: Interaction of pefloxacin and enoxacin with the human cytochrome P450 enzyme CYP1A2. Clin Pharmacol Ther 65:262–274, 1999

Kivisto KT, Lamberg TS, Kantola T, et al: Plasma buspirone concentrations are greatly increased by erythromycin and itraconazole. Clin Pharmacol Ther 62:348–354, 1997

Kivisto KT, Kantola T, Neuvonen PJ: Different effects of itraconazole on the pharmacokinetics of fluvastatin and lovastatin. Br J Clin Pharmacol 46:49–53, 1998

Kivisto KT, Lamberg TS, Neuvonen PJ: Interactions of buspirone with itraconazole and rifampicin: effects on the pharmacokinetics of the active 1-(2-pyrimidinyl)-piperazine metabolite of buspirone. Pharmacol Toxicol 84:94–97, 1999

Kreek MJ, Garfield JW, Gutjahr CL, et al: Rifampin induced methadone withdrawal. N Engl J Med 294:1104–1106, 1976

Larsen JT, Hansen LL, Spigset O, et al: Fluvoxamine is a potent inhibitor of tacrine metabolism in vivo. Eur J Clin Pharmacol 55:375–382, 1999

Lazar JD, Wilner KD: Drug interactions with fluconazole. Rev Infect Dis 12 (suppl 3):S327–S333, 1990

Liaudet L, Buclin T, Jaccard C, et al: Severe ergotism associated with interaction between ritonavir and ergotamine. BMJ 318:771, 1999

Lomaestro BM, Piatek MA: Update on drug interactions with azole antifungal agents. Ann Pharmacother 32:915–928, 1998

Luurila H, Olkkola KT, Neuvonen PJ: Interaction between erythromycin and the benzodiazepines diazepam and flunitrazepam. Pharmacol Toxicol 78:117–122, 1996

Mandell GL, Bennett JE, Dolin R (eds): Principles and Practice of Infectious Diseases. Philadelphia, PA, Churchill Livingstone, 2000, pp 404–422

Markowitz JS, Gill HS, Devane CL, et al: Fluoroquinolone inhibition of clozapine metabolism (letter). Am J Psychiatry 154:881, 1997

Merry C, Mulcahy F, Barry M, et al: Saquinavir interaction with midazolam: pharmacokinetic considerations when prescribing protease inhibitors for patients with HIV disease. AIDS 11:268–269, 1997

Mizuki Y, Fujiwara I, Yamaguchi T: Pharmacokinetic interactions related to the chemical structures of fluoroquinolones. J Antimicrob Chemother 37 (suppl A):41–55, 1996

Neuvonen PJ, Kantola T, Kivisto KT: Simvastatin but not pravastatin is very susceptible to interaction with the CYP3A4 inhibitor itraconazole. Clin Pharmacol Ther 63:332–341, 1998

Olkkola KT, Aranko K, Luurila H, et al: A potentially hazardous interaction between erythromycin and midazolam. Clin Pharmacol Ther 53:298–305, 1993

Ouellet D, Hsu A, Qian J, et al: Effect of ritonavir on the pharmacokinetics of ethinyl oestradiol in healthy female volunteers. Br J Clin Pharmacol 46:111–116, 1998

Piscitelli SC, Kress DR, Bertz RJ, et al: The effect of ritonavir on the pharmacokinetics of meperidine and normeperidine. Pharmacotherapy 20:549–553, 2000a

Piscitelli SC, Burstein AH, Chaitt D, et al: Indinavir concentrations and St John's wort. Lancet 355:547–548, 2000b

Pollak PT, Sketris IS, MacKenzie SL, et al: Delirium probably induced by clarithromycin in a patient receiving fluoxetine. Ann Pharmacother 29:486–488, 1995

Preston SL, Postelnick M, Purdy BD, et al: Drug interactions in HIV-positive patients initiated on protease inhibitor therapy. AIDS 12:228–230, 1998

Quinupristin/Dalfopristin. The Medical Letter 41:109–110, 1999

Rapp RP: Pharmacokinetics and pharmacodynamics of intravenous and oral azithromycin: enhanced tissue activity and minimal drug interactions. Ann Pharmacother 32:785–793, 1998

Robson RA: The effects of quinolones on xanthine pharmacokinetics. Am J Med 92:22S–25S, 1992

Rubenstein E, Prokocimer P, Talbot GH: Safety and tolerability of quinupristin/dalfopristin: administration guidelines. J Antimicrob Chemother 44 (suppl A):37–46, 1999

Self TH, Chrisman CR, Baciewicz AM, et al: Isoniazid drug and food interactions. Am J Med Sci 317:304–311, 1999

Sovner R, Fogelman S: Ketoconazole therapy for atypical depression. J Clin Psychiatry 57:227–228, 1996

Spicer ST, Liddle C, Chapman JR, et al: The mechanism of cyclosporine toxicity induced by clarithromycin. Br J Clin Pharmacol 43:194–196, 1997

Spina E, Pisani F, Perucca E: Clinically significant pharmacokinetic drug interactions with carbamazepine: an update. Clin Pharmacokinet 31:198–214, 1996

Sporanox package insert. Titusville, NJ, Janssen Pharmaceutica Products, LP, 2000

Strayhorn VA, Baciewicz AM, Self TH: Update on rifampin drug interactions, III. Arch Intern Med 157:2453–2458, 1997

Sustiva package insert. Wilmington, DE, DuPont Pharmaceuticals, 1999

Temple ME, Nahata MC: Rifapentine: its role in the treatment of tuberculosis. Ann Pharmacother 33:1203–1210, 1999

Tokinaga N, Kondo T, Kaneko S, et al: Hallucinations after a therapeutic dose of benzodiazepine hypnotics with co-administration of erythromycin. Psychiatry Clin Neurosci 50:337–339, 1996

Tseng AL, Foisy MM: Management of drug interactions in patients with HIV. Ann Pharmacother 31:1040–1058, 1997

Viagra package insert. New York, NY, Pfizer, Inc, 2000

Villikka K, Kivisto KT, Luurila H, et al: Rifampin reduces plasma concentrations and effects of zolpidem. Clin Pharmacol Ther 62:629–634, 1997

Viramune package insert. Ridgefield, CT, Boehringer Ingelheim Pharmaceuticals, Inc, and Roxane Laboratories, 1996

von Moltke LL, Greenblatt DJ, Grassi JM, et al: Protease inhibitors as inhibitors of human cytochromes P450: high risk associated with ritonavir. J Clin Pharmacol 38:106–111, 1998

Watkins JS, Polk RE, Stotka JL: Drug interactions of macrolides: emphasis on dirithromycin. Ann Pharmacother 31:349–356, 1997

Yasui N, Otani K, Kaneko S, et al: A kinetic and dynamic study of oral alprazolam with and without erythromycin in humans: in vivo evidence for the involvement of CYP3A4 in alprazolam metabolism. Clin Pharmacol Ther 59:514–519, 1996

Zhao XJ, Koyama E, Ishizaki T: An in vitro study on the metabolism and possible drug interactions of rokitamycin, a macrolide antibiotic, using human liver microsomes. Drug Metab Dispos 27:776–785, 1999

13

NEUROLOGY

Neurology and psychiatry share many pharmacological treatments and oftentimes patients. The use of tricyclic antidepressants and selective serotonin reuptake inhibitors for poststroke depression, tricyclic antidepressants for migraine prophylaxis, anticholinesterases for dementia, and the overlapping psychiatric and neurological uses of antiepileptic drugs are just a few examples. The antiepileptics are associated with significant P450-mediated interactions, both as substrates and as potent inducers of enzymes. In this chapter, we cover antiepileptic agents in detail and then briefly review antiparkinsonian drugs, cholinesterase inhibitors for dementia, and ergots as substrates that are sometimes affected by P450 inhibitors and inducers.

> Reminder: In this chapter, only P450-mediated drug interactions are discussed. Interactions due to displaced protein-binding, alterations in absorption or excretion, and pharmacodynamic interactions are not covered.

■ ANTIEPILEPTIC DRUGS

Phenobarbital was noted to be efficacious for seizure control in 1912, phenytoin was marketed in 1938, and valproate was marketed in 1968. The metabolism of these three drugs was and in some ways remains a mystery. Drugs developed after the late 1980s have undergone human liver microsome studies and some in vivo testing with probes. Unfortunately, many older drugs, being off patent, have not been reevaluated with this new technology. The hepatic enzymes involved in phenobarbital and valproate metabolism have been deduced from their in vivo drug interactions, and the older literature is sometimes confusing. Phenytoin has been relatively well studied, having become a probe drug for 2C9 and 2C19. We discuss in detail the antiepileptics with inducing or inhibiting potential and those with narrow therapeutic windows that may be easily affected by P450-active drugs. Gabapentin has no P450 metabolism and is excreted by the kidney unchanged. Oxcarbazepine is new to the U.S. market and has an interesting P450 interaction profile.

General Drug Interactions

Barbiturates

Primidone is metabolized to phenobarbital, and phenobarbital is metabolized at 2C9, 2C19, and 2E1 (Tanaka 1999). The metabolism of phenobarbital may be *inhibited* by potent inhibitors of these enzymes, including felbamate (Reidenberg et al. 1995) and valproic acid (Bernus et al. 1994). It would be expected that potent 2C9 and 2C19 inhibitors such as fluvoxamine and the pan-inhibitor ritonavir would also inhibit the metabolism of phenobarbital and other barbiturates.

Barbiturates have been known for decades to be metabolic *inducers*. All barbiturates induce enzyme metabolism and are "pan-inducers," meaning that they affect all inducible enzymes. In a 1993 prospective study of neonates in the intensive care setting, Yoshida et al. found that when phenobarbital was given to patients with therapeutic phenytoin levels, their phenytoin levels dropped significantly shortly after phenobarbital was added. Phenobarbital induces the metabolism of oral contraceptives as well (see Chapter 10). Shane-McWhorter et al. (1998) reported levonorgestrel failure in an epileptic patient with a levonorgestrel implant who became pregnant twice while on phenobarbital.

Psychotropics are greatly effected by phenobarbital. von Bahr et al. (1998) administered nortriptyline for 4 weeks to six healthy volunteers, adding phenobarbital on days 8–21. Nortriptyline levels decreased after 2 days of phenobarbital administration, and clear-

■ ANTIEPILEPTIC DRUGS

Drug	Metabolism	Enzyme(s) or route inhibited	Enzyme(s) induced
Carbamazepine	3A4, 2C9, 1A2	None known	**3A4**[a], phase II
Ethosuximide	3A4	None known	None known
Felbamate	3A4, 2E1	2C19	3A4
Lamotrigine	Phase II	None known	None known
Levetiracetam	None known	None known	None known
Oxcarbazepine	None known	None known	3A4
Phenobarbital	Complex, involves phase I and II	3A4,[b] ?phase II	**3A4**,[a] ?2D6, phase II
Phenytoin	2C9, 2C19, 2E1, phase II	None known	**3A4**,[a] phase II
Primidone	Complex, involves phase I and II	3A4,[b] ?phase II	**3A4**,[a] ?2D6, phase II
Tiagabine	3A4	None known	None known
Topiramate	Phase II	None known	?3A4
Valproate	Complex, phase II, 2C9, 2C19, 2A6	2D6[b], phase II	2C9, 2C19, phase II

Note. Gabapentin is excreted unchanged in urine.
[a]Potent (bold type).
[b]Moderate.
[c]Mild.

ance of nortriptyline increased twofold. These authors also reminded us that the decrease in nortriptyline levels was faster than the increase after phenobarbital was stopped. Induction of 3A4 and 2C9 is the probable mechanism of this interaction. Spina et al. (1996b) compared desipramine metabolism in eight epileptic patients and eight control subjects who were all extensive metabolizers at 2D6. The epileptic patients were on steady-state phenobarbital therapy. A single dose of desipramine was administered to all, and the epileptic patients had a lower area under the curve (AUC) and maximal drug concentration (C_{max}) and shorter elimination half-life than the healthy control subjects. Clozapine metabolism was also shown to be induced by phenobarbital in a study comparing schizophrenic patients and healthy control subjects (Facciola et al. 1998).

Carbamazepine

Carbamazepine is the most widely used antiepileptic, with several off-label uses. The drug induces its own metabolism, both phase I and II. The half-life decreases from 35.6 to 20.9 hours after multiple doses, with the steady-state concentration reducing 50% after 3 weeks. Carbamazepine also induces the metabolism of other drugs, particularly those dependent on 3A4 for metabolism, yet it has been found to induce 1A2 as well, affecting the metabolism of caffeine (Parker et al. 1998). Carbamazepine has been shown to reduce the half-life and increase oral clearance of ethosuximide (Giaccone et al. 1996). Potent inducers of 3A4, such as rifampin or phenobarbital, may decrease carbamazepine serum levels.

The epoxidation of carbamazepine occurs at 3A4, its major metabolic pathway, 2C9 and 1A2 being minor pathways (Spina et al. 1996a). Therefore, potent inhibitors of 3A4 (ketoconazole, ritonavir, erythromycin, and clarithromycin) may increase carbamazepine levels beyond the therapeutic window (Spina et al. 1997). Fluconazole, a mild to moderate inhibitor of 3A4 (and usually recommended as the safest azole antifungal with respect to drug interactions), has been noted in a few case reports to increase carbamazepine concentrations (Nair and Morris 1999), being a potent inhibitor of 2C9.

Oxcarbazepine

Oxcarbazepine was developed to sidestep the problems associated with carbamazepine (see "Carbamazepine" section above). Oxcarbazepine is supposed to have a low level of hepatic induction. It has been noted that when patients are switched from carbamazepine to oxcarbazepine while taking other P450-dependent antiepileptic drugs, the other antiepileptic drugs may reach toxic levels after 2–4 weeks of oxcarbazepine. These increased drug levels occur after the carbamazepine-induced enzymes return to normal functioning (Tecoma 1999).

Oxcarbazepine seems not to be affected itself by potent inhibitors of P450 enzymes like erythromycin and cimetidine. Tecoma (1999) suggested that oxcarbazepine dosing may need to be increased if it is coadministered with potent P450-inducing drugs.

Oxcarbazepine does seem to *induce* P450 metabolism of ethinyl estradiol (EE) and levonorgestrel, probably at 3A4. Fattore et al. (1999) studied 16 healthy women over two menstrual cycles in a randomized, double-blind, crossover study. AUC, peak plasma concentrations, and half-lives of EE and levonorgestrel were decreased with oxcarbazepine coadministration. Breakthrough bleeding occurred with these combinations, but these authors found no surge in progesterone levels (ovulation).

Oxcarbazepine may have better side-effect, autoinduction, and toxicity profiles than carbamazepine, but its P450 induction profile may be comparable to the other inducing antiepileptic drugs—carbamazepine, phenytoin, and the barbiturates (Armstrong and Cozza 2000).

Felbamate

Because of its potential for hepatotoxicity and producing aplastic anemia, felbamate is reserved for treatment of refractory seizures. The drug is metabolized by 3A4 and 2E1 and has been induced by carbamazepine, phenytoin, and phenobarbital. Felbamate does not seem to be easily inhibited by 3A4 inhibitors such as erythromycin. In vitro and in vivo, this agent has been shown to inhibit 2C19, decreasing phenytoin clearance and increasing serum levels. Felbamate induces 3A4, reducing stable carbamazepine levels and concentrations of the progestin gestodene (Glue et al. 1997).

Lamotrigine

Lamotrigine is mostly metabolized by glucuronic acid conjugation but is also affected by enzyme-inducing and enzyme-inhibiting drugs, the mechanisms of which have not been fully evaluated. Valproic acid increases lamotrigine's half-life and seems to decrease the clearance of lamotrigine, necessitating a reduction in lamotrigine dose when the two drugs are coadministered. The mechanism for this interaction seems to be inhibition of phase II glucuronidation. Carbamazepine, phenytoin, phenobarbital, and primidone all decrease lamotrigine's half-life and increase its oral clearance (Bottiger et al. 1999; Matsuo 1999). Lamotrigine itself seems to cause no clinically significant changes in other antiepileptics when added to regimens of patients in whom drug concentrations have achieved a steady state (i.e., it neither induces nor inhibits metabolism on its own). Lamotrigine is associated with multiorgan failure (rarely) and with severe skin rashes, so careful dosing in patients receiving valproic acid or other inhibiting drugs is prudent.

Levetiracetam

Levetiracetam was developed in the late 1990s as add-on therapy for patients with refractory complex partial seizures. The agent has a limited metabolism in humans, with 66% of the dose excreted in the urine unchanged. In vitro studies indicate that levetiracetam is not metabolized by P450, nor does the drug inhibit or induce P450 enzymes. In vivo studies involving healthy volunteers and epileptic patients are needed to confirm the favorable P450-mediated interaction profile.

Phenytoin

The study of phenytoin has been complicated. Phenytoin is highly protein bound and can displace or be displaced by many other drugs. In addition, because phenytoin is metabolized at 2C9 and 2C19, genetic polymorphisms affect the metabolism of this drug, which was not known to early investigators, to whom the reasons for such varying individual responses were a mystery. Drugs that inhibit 2C9 and 2C19 (see tables in Chapters 7 and 8) will "convert" extensive metabolizers to poor metabolizers and increase phenytoin levels in those individuals, while not apparently slowing the metabolism in persons who are already poor metabolizers. Potent 2C9 inhibitors include fluvoxamine and fluconazole; fluoxetine is a moderate inhibitor. Potent inhibitors of 2C19 include fluvoxamine, ticlopidine, and omeprazole; again, fluoxetine is a moderate inhibitor. Rifamycins induce phenytoin metabolism.

Phenytoin itself is a potent inducer of 3A4 and phase II metabolism, and, when added to stable 3A4-dependent drug regimens, phenytoin may decrease the serum levels of these drugs after the first few weeks, necessitating dose adjustment.

Tiagabine

Tiagabine is metabolized at 3A4 and is susceptible to induction by other antiepileptic drugs that induce this enzyme. Tiagabine administration in patients taking valproic acid has been associated with a mild decrease in valproic acid levels, the mechanism of which is unclear (Brodie 1995; Gustavson et al. 1998); in general, however, tiagabine is not considered a P450 inhibitor or inducer (Kalviainen 1998).

Valproic Acid

Valproic acid is highly protein bound and is involved in many interactions because of protein-binding displacement. The agent also is extensively metabolized in the liver to 50 or more metabolites (Pisani 1992). Valproic acid metabolism is induced by carbamazepine, phenobarbital, primidone, and phenytoin, resulting in an increase in total valproate clearance of 30%–85%. When valproic acid is induced, the production of a toxic metabolite, 4-ene-valproic acid, is increased. Levels of this toxic metabolite are not measured in routine valproic acid laboratory tests. The metabolite 4-ene-valproic acid is a suspect in the hepatotoxicity of valproic acid. The risk factors for valproic acid–induced hepatotoxicity are male gender, age less than 2 years, neurological disease (other than seizures), and treatment with a P450-inducing medication in conjunction with valproic acid therapy. Sadeque et al. (1997) studied 4-ene-valproic acid reactions in vitro. These researchers' findings suggest that it is *not*

3A4 that is responsible for the increase in toxic metabolite but rather that 2C9 and 2A6 catalyze terminal desaturation of valproic acid. Valproic acid is a mild to moderate inhibitor of 2D6 as well as a moderate inducer of 2C9, 2C19, and phase II metabolism.

Psychotropic Drug Interactions

P450 Induction

Carbamazepine, phenytoin, phenobarbital, and felbamate may all decrease drug levels by induction, particularly if the other drug is metabolized primarily by 3A4. Therefore, tricyclic antidepressants, clozapine, and the triazolobenzodiazepines may need dosage adjustments when administered along with these 3A4 inducers (Facciola et al. 1998). Olanzapine is induced by carbamazepine, even though olanzapine is not dependent on 3A4 for metabolism. Carbamazepine has been shown to induce 1A2 in vitro and in vivo (Lucas et al. 1998).

Hesslinger et al. (1999) studied the effects of carbamazepine and valproic acid on the pharmacokinetics of haloperidol in a controlled clinical trial. Subjects with schizophrenia or schizoaffective disorder received haloperidol alone, haloperidol and carbamazepine, or haloperidol and valproic acid. The haloperidol dose remained stable, and the antiepileptic agents were adjusted to therapeutic levels. Carbamazepine significantly decreased plasma haloperidol levels, producing worsened clinical symptoms compared with symptoms in patients taking haloperidol only. Valproic acid had no effect on haloperidol levels or clinical outcome. The authors suggested that haloperidol taken with carbamazepine may result in treatment failure if haloperidol doses are not increased.

P450 Inhibition

Fluvoxamine and fluoxetine are inhibitors of 2C9 and 2C19, and phenytoin levels have increased with the addition of fluoxetine. Shad and Preskorn (1999) reported a decrease in phenytoin levels and effect when fluoxetine was discontinued.

Valproic acid is a moderate inhibitor. In an open-label, sequential, two-period study involving healthy volunteers, valproic acid increased amitriptyline serum levels by 31% and increased combined tricyclic antidepressant levels 19% higher than baseline (Wong et al. 1996).

Summary

Antiepileptic drugs are generally inducers of P450 enzymes and can therefore reduce the efficacy of coadministered drugs, particularly oral contraceptives (Guberman 1999) and drugs in combination antiepileptics. Carbamazepine and many other agents are metabolized at 3A4 and may reach toxic levels when administered with potent inhibitors such as erythromycin, ritonavir, or grapefruit juice. Phenytoin is metabolized at 2C9 and 2C19, so coadministration with drugs such as fluvoxamine and ticlopidine may lead to phenytoin toxicity. Valproic acid is a drug with a complicated metabolism and the potential for hepatotoxicity; therefore, serum levels of all coadministered medications with the potential for toxicity should be carefully monitored, as should levels of liver-associated enzymes.

■ ANTIPARKINSONIAN DRUGS

A *MEDLINE* search and a review of available literature revealed no reports of clinically significant P450-mediated interactions associated with antiparkinsonian drugs. The data presented in the table below are derived from in vitro studies of these drugs.

■ CHOLINESTERASE INHIBITORS

General and Psychotropic Drug Interactions

Donepezil

The manufacturer of donepezil studied this drug extensively in healthy volunteers and found no significant interactions between donepezil and theophylline, digoxin, warfarin, cimetidine, and ketoconazole (Tiseo et al. 1998). The lack of significant inhibition of donepezil with coadministration of the potent 3A4 inhibitor keto-

172

■ ANTIPARKINSONIAN DRUGS

Drug	Metabolism	Enzyme(s) inhibited	Enzyme(s) induced
Catechol *O*-methyltransferase inhibitors			
Tolcapone	Glucuronidation	2C19[d]	None known
Dopamine agonists			
Bromocriptine	3A4	2D6,[b] 3A4[b]	None known
Carbidopa-levodopa	None known	None known	None known
Pergolide	3A4	3A4[c]	None known
Pramipexole	Renal excretion	None known	None known
Ropinirole	1A2, 3A4	2D6,[b] 1A2[c]	None known
Selegiline/deprenyl	2D6, others	None known	None known

[a]Potent (bold type).
[b]Moderate.
[c]Mild.
[d]Mild—clinically insignificant.

■ CHOLINESTERASE INHIBITORS

Drug	Metabolism site(s)	Enzyme(s) inhibited	Enzyme(s) induced
Donepezil	2D6, 3A4	None known	None known
Tacrine	1A2	1A2	None known

conazole is most likely due to the fact that donepezil is primarily metabolized at 2D6. Carrier (1999) reported a case of worsened cholinergic side effects when paroxetine was administered with donepezil, most likely due to the selective serotonin reuptake inhibitor's 2D6 and moderate 3A4 inhibition. Donepezil is not a known inhibitor or inducer of any enzymes.

Tacrine

Tacrine is extensively metabolized by the liver, with extensive first-pass metabolism by 1A2. The agent competitively inhibits theophylline at 1A2 and has been shown to increase theophylline levels, leading to toxicity (Fontana et al. 1998; Madden et al. 1995). Tacrine is inhibited by the potent 1A2 inhibitor fluvoxamine, which in healthy volunteers increased the C_{max} and AUC significantly and caused the cholinergic side effects nausea, vomiting, diarrhea, and diaphoresis. Fluvoxamine inhibition is being studied as a mechanism for preventing tacrine hepatotoxicity. 1A2 mediates the production of a quinone methide via a 7-hydroxytacrine intermediate, which may be the pathway that makes the hepatotoxic substance. If it is found that fluvoxamine or another potent inhibitor can slow or prevent the production of this hepatotoxin, yet allow for the therapeutic effect of tacrine, the morbidity associated with tacrine could be greatly lessened. Further study is needed in this area (Becquemont et al. 1997; Larsen et al. 1999). Tacrine levels have also been increased by cimetidine (Forgue et al. 1996). Hormone replacement therapy containing levonorgestrel and estradiol has increased plasma tacrine concentrations as well, which may also lead to worsened cholinergic side effects in patients administered hormone replacement therapy for treatment of Alzheimer's disease or for osteoporosis prevention, but further study is needed (Laine et al. 1999).

■ ERGOTAMINES

Ergot derivatives are used as vasodilators in migraine treatment and, more recently, in the treatment of dementia. Ergotamines are metabolized at 3A4 and are mild to moderate inhibitors of 3A4 as well. Potent 3A4 inhibitors, particularly the macrolide antibiotics, have caused frank ergotism in patients. Horowitz et al. (1996) reported that a patient receiving clarithromycin therapy developed lingual ischemia after taking a 2-mg dose of ergotamine tartrate. Nicergoline, an ergot not yet available in the United States, has been used for the treatment of dementia in Europe. This agent seems to be metabolized by 2D6, as determined in studies involving healthy volunteers (Bottinger et al. 1996). Studies of this drug in combination with potent 2D6 inhibitors have not yet been conducted.

■ REFERENCES

Armstrong SC, Cozza KL: Consultation-liaison psychiatry drug-drug interactions update: drug interactions with antiepileptic drugs carbamazepine and oxcarbazepine. Psychosomatics 4:541–543, 2000

Becquemont L, Ragueneau I, LeBot MA, et al: Influence of the CYP1A2 inhibitor fluvoxamine on tacrine pharmacokinetics in humans. Clin Pharmacol Ther 61:619–627, 1997

Bernus I, Dickinson RG, Hooper WD, et al: Inhibition of phenobarbitone *N*-glucosidation by valproate. Br J Clin Pharmacol 38:411–416, 1994

Bloomer JC, Clarke SE, Chenery RJ: In vitro identification of the P450 enzymes responsible for the metabolism of ropinirole. Drug Metab Dispos 25:840–844, 1997

Bottiger Y, Dostert P, Benedetti MS, et al: Involvement of CYP2D6 but not CYP2C19 in nicergoline metabolism in humans. Br J Clin Pharmacol 42:707–711, 1996

Bottiger Y, Svensson JO, Stahle L: Lamotrigine drug interactions in a TDM material. Ther Drug Monit 21:171–174, 1999

Brodie MJ: Tiagabine pharmacology in profile. Epilepsia 36 (suppl 6):S7–S9, 1995

Carrier L: Donepezil and paroxetine: possible drug interaction (letter). J Am Geriatr Soc 47:1037, 1999

Donahue S, Flockhart DA, Abernethy DR: Ticlopidine inhibits phenytoin clearance. Clin Pharmacol Ther 66:563–568, 1999

Facciola G, Avenoso A, Spina E, et al: Inducing effect of phenobarbital on clozapine metabolism in patients with chronic schizophrenia. Ther Drug Monit 20:628–630, 1998

Fattore C, Cipolla G, Gatti G, et al: Induction of ethinylestradiol and levonorgestrel metabolism by oxcarbazepine in healthy women. Epilepsia 40:783–787, 1999

Fontana RJ, deVries TM, Woolf TF, et al: Caffeine based measures of CYP1A2 activity correlate with oral clearance of tacrine in patients with Alzheimer's disease. Br J Clin Pharmacol 46:221–228, 1998

Forgue ST, Reece PA, Sedman AJ, et al: Inhibition of tacrine metabolism by cimetidine. Clin Pharmacol Ther 59:444–449, 1996

Giaccone M, Bartoli A, Gatti G, et al: Effect of enzyme inducing anticonvulsants on ethosuximide pharmacokinetics in epileptic patients. Br J Clin Pharmacol 41:575–579, 1996

Glue P, Banfield CR, Perhach JL, et al: Pharmacokinetic interactions with felbamate: in vitro–in vivo correlation. Clin Pharmacokinet 33:214–224, 1997

Grace JM, Kinter MT, Macdonald TL: Atypical metabolism of deprenyl and its enantiomer, (S)-(+)-N,alpha-dimethyl-N-propynylphenethylamine by cytochrome P450 2D6. Chem Res Toxicol 7:286–290, 1994

Guberman A: Hormonal contraception with epilepsy. Neurology 53:S38–S40, 1999

Gustavson LE, Sommerville KW, Boellner SW, et al: Lack of a clinically significant pharmacokinetic drug interaction between tiagabine and valproate. Am J Ther 5:73–79, 1998

Hesslinger B, Normann C, Langosch JM, et al: Effects of carbamazepine and valproate on haloperidol plasma levels and on psychopathologic outcome in schizophrenic patients. J Clin Psychopharmacol 19:310–315, 1999

Horowitz RS, Dart RC, Gomez HF: Clinical ergotism with lingual ischemia induced by clarithromycin-ergotamine interaction. Arch Intern Med 156:456–458, 1996

Kalviainen R: Tiagabine: a new therapeutic option for people with intellectual disability and partial epilepsy. J Intellect Disabil Res 42 (suppl 1):63–67, 1998

Laine K, Palovaara S, Tapanainen P, et al: Plasma tacrine concentrations are significantly increased by concomitant hormone replacement therapy. Clin Pharmacol Ther 66:602–628, 1999

Larsen JT, Hansen LL, Spigset O, et al: Fluvoxamine is a potent inhibitor of tacrine metabolism in vivo. Eur J Clin Pharmacol 55:375–382, 1999

Lucas RA, Gilfillan DJ, Bergstrom RF: A pharmacokinetic interaction between carbamazepine and olanzapine: observations on possible mechanism. Eur J Clin Pharmacol 54:639–643, 1998

Madden S, Spaldin V, Park BK: Clinical pharmacokinetics of tacrine. Clin Pharmacokinet 28:449–457, 1995

Matsuo F: Lamotrigine. Epilepsia 40 (suppl 5):S30–S36, 1999

Mirapex package insert. Kalamazoo, MI, Pharmacia & Upjohn, Inc, 1997

Nair DR, Morris HH: Potential fluconazole-induced carbamazepine toxicity. Ann Pharmacother 33:790–792, 1999

Parker AC, Pritchard P, Preston T, et al: Induction of CYP1A2 activity by carbamazepine in children using the caffeine breath test. Br J Clin Pharmacol 45:176–178, 1998

Pisani F: Influence of co-medication on the metabolism of valproate. Pharmaceutisch Weekblad. Scientific Edition 14:108–113, 1992

Reidenberg P, Glue P, Banfield CR, et al: Effects of felbamate on the pharmacokinetics of phenobarbital. Clin Pharmacol Ther 58:279–287, 1995

Sadeque AJM, Fisher MB, Korzekwa KR, et al: Human CYP2C9 and CYP2A6 mediate formation of the hepatotoxin 4-ene-valproic acid. J Pharmacol Exp Ther 283:698–703, 1997

Schmider J, Greenblatt DJ, von Moltke LL, et al: Inhibition of CYP2C9 by selective serotonin reuptake inhibitors in vitro: studies of phenytoin p-hydroxylation. Br J Clin Pharmacol 44:495–498, 1997

Shad MU, Preskorn SH: Drug-drug interaction in reverse: possible loss of phenytoin efficacy as a result of fluoxetine discontinuation. J Clin Psychopharmacol 19:471–472, 1999

Shane-McWhorter L, Cerveny JD, MacFarlane LL, et al: Enhanced metabolism of levonorgestrel during phenobarbital treatment and resultant pregnancy. Pharmacotherapy 18:1360–1364, 1998

Spina E, Pisani F, Perucca E: Clinically significant pharmacokinetic drug interactions with carbamazepine. Clin Pharmacokinet 31:198–214, 1996a

Spina E, Avenoso A, Campo GM, et al: Phenobarbital induces the 2-hydroxylation of desipramine. Ther Drug Monit 18:60–64, 1996b

Spina E, Arena D, Scordo MG, et al: Elevation of plasma carbamazepine concentrations by ketoconazole in patients with epilepsy. Ther Drug Monit 19:535–538, 1997

Tanaka E: Clinically significant pharmacokinetic drug interactions between antiepileptic drugs. J Clin Pharm Ther 24:87–92, 1999

Tasmar package insert. Nutley, NJ, Roche Laboratories Inc, 1998

Tecoma ES: Oxcarbazepine. Epilepsia 40 (suppl 5):S37–S46, 1999

Tiseo PJ, Perdomo CA, Friedhoff LT: Concurrent administration of donepezil HCl and cimetidine: assessment of pharmacokinetic changes following single and multiple doses. Br J Clin Pharmacol 46 (suppl 1):25–29, 1998 von Bahr C, Steiner E, Koike Y, et al: Time course of enzyme induction in humans: effect of pentobarbital on nortriptyline metabolism. Clin Pharmacol Ther 64:18–26, 1998

Wong SL, Cavanaugh J, Shi H, et al: Effects of divalproex sodium on amitriptyline and nortriptyline pharmacokinetics. Clin Pharmacol Ther 60: 48–53, 1996

Yoshida N, Oda Y, Nishi S, et al: Effect of barbiturate therapy on phenytoin pharmacokinetics. Crit Care Med 21:1514–1522, 1993

14

ONCOLOGY

Michael A. Cole, M.D.

The use of multiple drugs in oncology is commonplace. Antiemetics, antibiotics, analgesics, and even anticonvulsants all have the potential for adverse pharmacokinetic effects on antineoplastic agents. Little is known about the relationships between P450 enzymes and many of the older drugs used in oncology. Because antineoplastic agents have such narrow therapeutic windows, small changes in the pharmacokinetics of these drugs may have serious adverse effects, such as cytopenias and mucositis.

Specific enzyme studies of many of the drugs used in oncology are lacking, because of the age of the drugs and because the toxicity of these agents usually prevents their use in in vivo pharmacokinetic drug studies. Another problem is that many anticancer drugs are administered in combination regimens, making identification of some interactions and effects difficult. Much of the known metabolism, inhibition, and induction effects of these drugs were determined in in vitro cell and tissue culture studies. Findings of in vitro studies may not correlate with the in vivo use of any given drug, but these findings should be given consideration (McLeod 1998).

In pediatric patients, isoforms of enzymes are known to develop at different rates, with some enzymes not being present at all and others not present in amounts equivalent to those in adults. For example, fetal liver microsomes have approximately 1% of adult activity levels, and these levels increase to an average of 70% by day 7 of extrauterine life. The majority of the data in this chapter can be extrapolated to apply to children older than 10–12 years, but a more thorough review of developmental pharmacokinetics in the pediatric subpopulation is warranted. A good review can be found in a report by Leeder and Kearns (1997).

In this chapter, the known P450-mediated interactions of many classes of chemotherapeutic drugs, including immunomodulators, are reviewed. Unless specific reference is made to a particular drug, no P450-mediated effects were identified by *MEDLINE* searches. For many drugs, I needed to expand the search to include animal studies. I have attempted to cover the classes and drugs that are used routinely in oncology practice, and I did not focus on new and investigational agents. (For information on antiemetic drugs, see Chapter 15.)

> Reminder: In this chapter, only P450-mediated interactions are discussed. Interactions due to displaced protein-binding, alterations in absorption or excretion, and pharmacodynamic interactions are not covered.

◼ ANTINEOPLASTIC DRUGS

Alkylating Agents

Alkylating agents are some of the more frequently used drugs in chemotherapy. The main effect of these drugs is the cross-linking of strands of DNA, resulting in breakage and cell death. Although cross-linking DNA strands works most effectively in cells that are actively proliferating, alkylating agents can damage cells during any phase of the cell cycle.

Busulfan

In a prospective study of high-dose busulfan pharmacokinetics, patients receiving prophylactic phenytoin had significantly higher clearance of busulfan than did patients receiving diazepam (Hassan et al. 1993). Subjects administered high-dose busulfan and no other medications had normal clearance rates. These authors did not comment on P450-mediated effects, but this finding strongly suggests induction of 3A4 by phenytoin, resulting in increased clearance of busulfan.

Cyclophosphamide, Ifosfamide, and Trofosfamide

Cyclophosphamide, ifosfamide, and trofosfamide are alkylating pro-drugs that require metabolism by P450 enzymes for antitumor activity. Studies have shown that the enzymes 2B1, 3A4, 2C9, and 2C19 are important for their metabolism. In a study by Chen et al. (1997), human breast cancer cells grown in mice were transfected with a gene for 2B1. Cytotoxicity was increased 15- to 20-fold in the breast cancer cells with this gene, compared with cells lacking the gene, which points to the possible effectiveness of gene therapy in certain types of cancer. Philip et al. (1999) also found, in a mouse model, that cyclophosphamide and ifosfamide were only cytotoxic to cells expressing the 2B1 or 3A4 enzymes.

Bohnenstengel and colleagues (1996) reported in vitro data showing that 3A4 is the enzyme that performs side-chain oxidation (*N*-dealkylation) of cyclophosphamide, resulting in the formation of chloroacetaldehyde, a potential neurotoxic agent. Although the likely toxicity of chloroacetaldehyde has not been disputed in the literature, there are no data to support in vivo reports of toxicity. The potential may exist for significant neurotoxicity during high-dose chemotherapy with cyclophosphamide or if standard doses are used in the presence of an inducer of 3A4. (See "Induction" in Chapter 3.)

Clinical anecdotes suggest that cyclophosphamide may induce its own metabolism and are supported by an in vitro study using human liver microsomes that showed that administration of either cyclophosphamide or ifosfamide results in increased production of several P450 enzymes, including 3A4 and 2C9 (T.K. Chang et al. 1997). The same study showed increased oxidation of cyclophosphamide and ifosfamide when the cultures were pretreated with dexamethasone, rifampin, or phenobarbital. This finding lends support to the concept of 3A4 metabolism of cyclophosphamide and ifosfamide, although the authors did not comment on levels of the neurotoxic metabolite chloroacetaldehyde.

Trofosfamide is a newer alkylating agent that also requires metabolism into its active metabolite. In in vitro assays of human liver microsomes, May-Manke et al. (1999) demonstrated metabolic activity at 3A4 and 2B6 without induction or inhibition of other enzymes. The lack of induction activity as seen with cyclophosphamide and ifosfamide might suggest that trofosfamide may have fewer drug-drug interactions, but there is no clinical evidence to support this at time of publication.

Carmustine and Lomustine

Little has been done to delineate specific enzymes that metabolize carmustine or lomustine. In 1975, Hill et al. demonstrated that carmustine is metabolized by microsomal enzymes in mouse liver and lungs. Levin et al. (1979) used a rat model to show that phenobarbital pretreatment increases clearance of carmustine and lomustine. These investigators also demonstrated that pretreatment with phenytoin or dexamethasone, both inducers of 3A4, did *not* affect clearance rates of either carmustine or lomustine. In their reports, Hill et al. (1975) and Levin et al. (1979) did not comment on specific P450 enzymes, but their data suggest that the responsible enzyme may be 2C9. Studies using human liver microsomes have not yet been repeated for either drug.

Streptozocin

P. Chang et al. (1976) reported decreased clearance of doxorubicin in patients who were also receiving streptozocin. The increased severity of side effects of doxorubicin in that study suggests hepatic dysfunction due to streptozocin, but no specific mention was made of P450 involvement.

Antimetabolites

Antimetabolites come in many forms, with multiple mechanisms of action. These drugs exert their cytotoxicity by acting as false substrates in multiple biochemical pathways. Nucleoside analogues are incorporated into newly formed DNA and result in termination of DNA growth. Other antimetabolite agents include enzyme inhibitors such as methotrexate, and all antimetabolites ultimately result in faulty DNA synthesis.

Methotrexate

Methotrexate is metabolized by oxidation but not via P450 (Chladek et al. 1997). A study using human liver microsomes showed that ethanol and acetaminophen, both inducers of 2E1, also increase levels of tumor necrosis factor–α, interleukin (IL)-6, and IL-8 (Neuman et al. 1999). These increases lead to reduced mitochondrial and cytosolic glutathione levels and an increase in the oxidative stress on cell cultures. These same cells were subsequently exposed to methotrexate and showed increased methotrexate-induced cytotoxicity and an increased rate of programmed cell death (apoptosis). This phenomenon is not specifically related to P450 enzymes but is important to consider, given known effects of cytokines on P450 activity. (See "Immunomodulators" later in this chapter.)

Fluorouracil

van Meerten et al. (1995) reviewed the then-available literature on drug-drug interactions and antineoplastic agents. They noted that both cimetidine and metronidazole inhibit the metabolism of fluorouracil, which suggests metabolism by P450 enzymes (3A4, 2D6). Interferon-α appears to decrease clearance of fluorouracil, a finding that is consistent with findings of studies showing interferon's effect on the downregulation of some P450 enzymes.

Taxanes

The taxanes are a group of compounds isolated from plants, specifically yews. Taxanes are antineoplastic because of their ability to stabilize cellular microtubules that are necessary during mitosis and to prevent their disassembly.

Docetaxel

Researchers used in vitro cell culture assays of human hepatocytes to measure the effect of several P450 enzymes on docetaxel metabolism and found oxidation predominantly at 3A4 and to a lesser extent at 3A5 (Shou et al. 1998). Clarke and Rivory (1999) reviewed the literature on docetaxel and suggested that patients with increased plasma bilirubin or transaminase levels experience a 12%–27% decrease in docetaxel clearance and should receive reduced doses.

Paclitaxel seems to increase serum levels of doxorubicin. An in vitro cell culture study examining the metabolism of paclitaxel and docetaxel found that oxidation of docetaxel was significantly inhibited by the 3A4 inhibitors ketoconazole and erythromycin and not by inhibitors of 2D6 such as quinidine (Royer et al. 1996). Steroids had no appreciable effect on the oxidation of docetaxel, although barbiturates have increased the rate of metabolism (Royer et al. 1996).

Paclitaxel

In vitro studies conducted with human liver microsomes and liver slices have shown that paclitaxel is metabolized by both 2C9 and 3A4 (Harris et al. 1994). In vivo data support this finding but demonstrate significant individual variability with regard to enzymes preferentially used. Results of the in vitro study by Rahman et al. (1994) suggest that 2C9 is the enzyme responsible for the principal metabolite.

In a prospective study, Jamis-Dow et al. (1997) evaluated the safety of concomitant administration of ketoconazole and paclitaxel in patients with ovarian cancer. The effect of ketoconazole on 3A4 was not sufficient to alter the metabolism of paclitaxel significantly. Jamis-Dow et al. (1997) noted that both may be administered simultaneously without dose adjustments. However, the investigators did not genotype their subjects. If all of the subjects had enough 2C9 activity, 3A4 inhibition by ketoconazole may not have affected paclitaxel's metabolism.

Methylprednisolone, a 3A4 inhibitor, was administered to a cancer patient for 14 days before administration of paclitaxel (Monsarrat et al. 1997). Measurement of the 3A4 metabolite of paclitaxel (dihydroxypaclitaxel) was performed via the patient's percutaneous biliary drain. Compared with two patients with percutaneous drains who had been previously studied by the authors, the patient pretreated with methylprednisolone had significantly increased levels of biliary dihydroxypaclitaxel.

Desai et al. (1998) tested multiple medications as inhibitors of the formation of the 2C9 and 3A4 metabolites of paclitaxel in in vitro human liver microsome preparations. These researchers found doxorubicin to be a significant inhibitor of the formation of the 3A4 metabolite and cyclosporine to be a significant inhibitor of the formation of the 2C9 metabolite. Both P450 metabolites were shown to be inhibited by tamoxifen, *R*-verapamil, and etoposide, but the authors suggested that this inhibition was more likely due to modulation of the multidrug resistance pump. Desai et al. (1998) made no references to the inhibition of specific enzymes by tamoxifen, *R*-verapamil, or etoposide. Paclitaxel was shown to significantly reduce the oxidation of docetaxel in vitro (Royer et al. 1996), suggesting that paclitaxel may inhibit 3A4 enzymes as well.

These data indicate that metabolism of paclitaxel occurs through both 3A4 and 2C9. In vitro data suggest multiple possible interactions, but few reports of in vivo studies or case reports support these data.

Vinca Alkaloids

Vinca alkaloids are another group of plant-derived drugs. Like the taxanes, vinca alkaloids disrupt cells in mitosis. These agents' mechanism of action is slightly different, in that vinca alkaloids inhibit microtubule assembly by binding to tubulin.

Vincristine

Chan (1998) conducted a thorough review of case reports and clinical studies of vinca alkaloids and their pharmacokinetics. All inhibitors of 3A4 reduce the metabolism of vincristine in vitro, and several case reports have indicated increased vincristine toxicity with concomitant use of 3A4 inhibitors, such as itraconazole and cyclosporine.

Drugs such as carbamazepine and phenytoin, known inducers of 3A4, have been shown to increase the metabolism of vincristine (used in combination with lomustine and procarbazine) in human volunteer subjects (Villikka et al. 1999). No studies have evaluated efficacy during concomitant administration.

Vinorelbine

Vinorelbine is a newer anticancer agent of the vinca alkaloid family. Kajita et al. (2000) used human liver microsome preparations to demonstrate that 3A4 is the main P450 enzyme responsible for metabolism of vinorelbine. The same study showed that high concentrations (100 μM) also inhibited 3A4 activity without inhibiting other P450 enzymes, but that this level is likely higher than that found in human plasma concentrations.

Topoisomerase Inhibitors

Successful replication of DNA is a complex process that is mediated by several enzymes. Tension is created in the DNA molecule during normal replication. Topoisomerase enzymes are crucial to making the DNA molecule flexible during replication. If topoisomerase enzymes are inhibited, this tension is not relieved, and DNA replication and cell reproduction cannot take place.

Etoposide and Teniposide

Etoposide and teniposide are partially metabolized by 3A4 (McLeod 1998; Relling et al. 1994). Cyclosporine's ability to decrease clearance of etoposide both in vitro and clinically has been noted in several reports, as has the need to decrease the dose of etoposide when these drugs are used concomitantly. Although both drugs are metabolized by 3A4, the need to decrease the dose is not due to a P450-mediated effect. Cyclosporine inhibits the multidrug resistance P-glycoprotein pump, causing cells to retain the etoposide for a longer period. Kusuhara and colleagues (1997) conducted a more extensive review of the multidrug resistance gene products and their clinical impact.

In a study involving patients with glioma and patients with small-cell lung cancer, the pharmacokinetic properties of etoposide were evaluated (Bagniewski et al. 1996). The area under the curve (AUC) was shown to be decreased in patients taking anticonvulsants and/or glucocorticoids. These data demonstrate that steroid- or anticonvulsant-inducible P450 enzymes are responsible for the increased clearance of etoposide, which is consistent with known effects of anticonvulsants and steroids on 3A4.

Irinotecan

Irinotecan is a topoisomerase inhibitor used in lung and colon cancers (Berkery 1997). Santos et al. (2000) used human liver microsome preparations to demonstrate that irinotecan is predominantly metabolized at 3A4 and to a varying degree at 3A5. No clinical drug interactions or adverse effects were identified in the literature.

Antitumor Antibiotics

Often referred to as anthracyclines, antitumor antibiotics are cytotoxic by a variety of mechanisms, but the underlying mechanism of these drugs is DNA damage. Some antitumor antibiotics lead to creation of free radicals that make double- and single-strand breaks in the DNA, whereas others in this group of agents cross-link the DNA strands and prevent replication.

Doxorubicin

Balis (1986) showed that P450 enzymes are involved in anthracycline metabolism, although no specific enzymes were delineated. Use of either phenytoin or phenobarbital increases the metabolism of doxorubicin. These data suggest that doxorubicin is partially metabolized at 3A4. There are multiple reports of in vitro studies of doxorubicin's effects on taxane metabolism, but no in vivo data could be found to demonstrate clinical relevance of this possible interaction.

Antiandrogens and Antiestrogens

The enzyme responsible for conversion of androgens (steroids) to estrogens in many human tissues is P450 aromatase, an important member of the P450 family that is also found in adipose, neural, and skin tissues. Because androgens (testosterone) and estrogens have such dramatic effects on some carcinomas (i.e., breast and prostate cancer), modulation of aromatase activity is a useful therapeutic modality.

Aminoglutethimide

Aminoglutethimide is a potent P450 aromatase inhibitor that is used in the treatment of metastatic breast cancer. Santner et al. (1984) studied preparations of human placental microsomes and other inhibitors of aromatase and noted that coadminstration of two aromatase inhibitors, aminoglutethimide and testololactone, produced an additive effect, evidenced by a decrease in aromatase activity greater than that seen with either agent alone. These investigators suggested that a dose reduction might be possible with aminoglutethimide, which would reduce possible side effects such as sedation, rash, and orthostatic hypotension.

Anastrozole

Anastrozole is another potent inhibitor of P450 aromatase and thus decreases the pro-growth effect of estrogen on breast cancer. Although no drug-drug interactions due to inhibition have been reported, in vitro studies using human liver microsomes have shown that anastrozole inhibits 1A2, 2C9, and 3A4 (Grimm and Dyroff 1997). Further discussion of the genetics and expression of aromatase can be found in a report by Simpson et al. (1997).

Flutamide

Flutamide is an androgen receptor antagonist that is often used in the treatment of prostate cancer. Using human liver microsome preparations, Shet et al. (1997) demonstrated that flutamide is metabolized to its primary metabolite by 1A2. A minor metabolite was formed by 3A4. This primary metabolite of flutamide, 2-hydroxyflutamide, is a more potent androgen receptor antagonist and can inhibit 1A2. No in vivo studies were found that focused on this phenomenon, and the clinical implications of 1A2 inhibition by 2-hydroxyflutamide cannot be adequately estimated from these few data.

Liarozole

Liarozole plays a role in chemotherapy for prostate and breast carcinomas. This agent inhibits not only P450 aromatase (Seidmon et al. 1995) but also CYP26, the P450 enzyme responsible for retinoic acid metabolism in humans (see "Retinoids" later in this chapter). In in vitro studies with human breast cancer cells, the enzyme induced by retinoic acid (CYP26) was significantly inhibited by liarozole, and the cytotoxicity of retinoic acid was enhanced by this effect (Sonneveld et al. 1998). Liarozole's ability to inhibit aromatase was used in investigational studies evaluating this effect on estrogen-dependent breast cancer patients. In a Phase II study, Goss et al. (1996) found that within 2 weeks of use, liarozole decreased plasma estrogen levels to an undetectable level. This finding raises hopes regarding the clinical usefulness of liarozole in breast cancer.

In a Phase III study, Debruyne et al. (1998) noted liarozole's decreasing of serum prostate-specific antigen levels in patients with metastatic prostate cancer. The investigators did not look specifically at P450-mediated effects but reported that liarozole decreased the amount of pain subjects experienced and also improved scores on objective assessments of overall quality of life. This study showed that an understanding of the effects of certain drugs on P450 enzymes can have significant benefits in clinical practice.

Tamoxifen

Tamoxifen is an older chemotherapy drug that works as an anti-estrogen, and tamoxifen's 4-hydroxylation metabolite is intrinsically 100 times more potent (Crewe et al. 1997). Human liver microsome studies have shown that tamoxifen is metabolized to a more active estrogen receptor antagonist by 4-hydroxylation at 2D6 (Dehal and Kupfer 1997). 3A4 also metabolizes tamoxifen by *N*-demethylation, but the metabolite is a less potent antiestrogen (Dehal and Kupfer 1997). Christians et al. (1996) determined that several drugs, including tamoxifen, may inhibit P450 metabolism of tacrolimus, a known 3A4 substrate. This finding strongly suggests that tamoxifen inhibits 3A4 and therefore its own metabolism.

A study of the interaction between rifampin and tamoxifen and toremifene found a marked reduction in the serum levels of tamoxifen and toremifene in patients also taking rifampin, a potent inducer of 3A4 (Kivisto et al. 1998).

Toremifene

Toremifene is metabolized at 3A4 and 1A. In vitro studies using human liver microsome preparations with known inhibitors showed that the majority (but not all) of the metabolites of the drug are created by these two isoforms (Berthou et al. 1994).

Vorozole

Vorozole is a new, third generation aromatase inhibitor that causes reversible inhibition of P450 aromatase (Goss 1998). Vorozole demonstrated significant response rates for inhibition of estradiol production in clinical Phase II trials with breast cancer patients (Goss 1998).

Miscellaneous Agents

Cisplatin and Other Platinum Agents

Platinum agents are the only heavy-metal compounds used for anti-neoplastic chemotherapy. Administration of these drugs results in covalent cross-linking of DNA, leading to an inability to replicate the DNA strands.

There are numerous reports in the literature that the use of cisplatin may decrease the serum levels of anticonvulsants, although none of these reports include comments on a specific mechanism. Although the platinum agents are predominantly cleared renally, there is a need for further exploration of their P450-mediated effects.

Ando and colleagues (1998) reported that JM216, a new agent and the only oral platinum compound to date, inhibited several P450 enzymes (3A4, 2C9, 1A1, 1A2, 2A6, 2E1, and 2D6). These authors provided no in vivo data and suggested that further studies need to be done.

Dacarbazine

Dacarbazine, a pro-drug like cyclophosphamide, was recently found to be metabolized to active forms by 1A1, 1A2, and 2E1. Inhibitors of these enzymes significantly inhibited the *N*-demethylation of dacarbazine in vitro (Reid et al. 1999).

Retinoids

Retinoic acid, a vitamin A derivative, plays an important role in the maintaining of normal cell growth and structure but has been shown to induce cell differentiation and development in both healthy and cancer cells, leading to earlier cell death. Retinoic acid was initially used only in cases of acute promyelocytic leukemia, but the drug has recently been administered to patients with other tumors. Early trials examined retinoic acid's effect on prostate cancers. More recent studies also evaluated its effect on breast carcinoma. Han and Choi (1996) found that retinoic acid was metabolized to 4- and 18-hydroxy metabolites. Retinoic acid induced its own metabolism, but human liver microsome assays of known inhibitors and inducers revealed no P450-mediated interactions.

All-*trans*-retinoic acid (ATRA) induces its metabolism. In a Phase II study of ATRA in prostate cancer patients, subjects who received 14 days of ATRA therapy had an 83% increase in activity of 2E1 as well as of Phase II *N*-acetyltransferase (Adedoyin et al. 1998). Subjects showed no appreciable differences in activity of 1A2, 2C19, 2D6, or 3A4. Krekels et al. (1997) performed in vitro assays with breast cancer cells and found that autoinduction of ATRA metabolism is dose dependent.

An in vitro study of several head and neck cancer cell lines showed that the oxidative catabolism of retinoids is inhibited by fluconazole (suggesting 3A4 or 2C9 catabolism) and induced by 13-*cis*-retinoic acid, 9-*cis*-retinoic acid, and retinal but not retinol (Kim et al. 1998). These findings were corroborated by Schwartz and colleagues (1995) in a prospective study involving patients with acute promyelocytic leukemia. However, Lee et al. (1995) found no differences in the AUC for ATRA with or without ketoconazole. The 3A4 enzyme may or may not be involved in ATRA's metabolism, but extrapolation of the data from these studies suggests that ATRA is metabolized by 2C9 to a much greater extent than by 3A4.

CYP26 is a P450 enzyme that has not been extensively characterized. Sonneveld et al. (1998) reviewed retinoid metabolism and its probable hydroxylation by CYP26, which is induced by ATRA. CYP26 was specific for the hydroxylation of ATRA only, not other isomers of retinoic acid. Although CYP26 is not a prominent P450 enzyme, its effect on retinoids is notable.

Steroids

Glucocorticoids are a common addition to many chemotherapy regimens. Using human hepatocyte cultures, Liddle (1998) showed that both dexamethasone and growth hormone (not a steroid per se) increased 3A4 activity (3A4 was the only enzyme on which the authors reported). This finding was corroborated by Christians et al. (1996) in further human liver microsome studies involving inhibition of tacrolimus metabolism.

■ IMMUNOMODULATORS

Much of the communication between cells, both healthy and diseased, is accomplished chemically. Cytokines are intercellular mediators that are released by cells in response to antigens or disease states in an effort to communicate with other cells, the immune system, or the body in general. Cytokines include but are not limited to chemical signals by interleukins, interferons, and other nonantibody proteins.

There has been a rapid increase in the number of drugs and synthetic antibodies routinely used in oncology as well as other areas of medicine. Many of these compounds are not metabolized by P450 enzymes but can have significant effects on the regulation of the level of activity of these enzymes. Additionally, P450 activity has been noted to fluctuate in many disease states, a concept supported by several in vitro human liver microsome studies showing changes in enzyme activity due to the effect of cytokines.

Interferon-α

Dorr (1993) reviewed available literature on the effects of interferon-α in multiple disease states and cited evidence that P450 enzymes, along with general cellular protein synthesis, are inhibited by interferon-α. In addition to reference provided by Leeder and Kearns (1997), Dorr (1993) noted increased clearance of theophylline in inflammatory disease states, suggesting possible 1A2 induction, although no reference was made to specific enzymes.

Cytokines and Interleukins

Gorski et al. (2000) briefly reviewed the decreases in P450 function observed with interleukin (IL)-6, tumor necrosis factor–α, and IL-1β therapy. In a study of IL-10 in healthy human volunteers, these investigators demonstrated a decrease in 3A4 activity without any effect on 1A2, 2C9, or 2D6. Observations in more clinical settings suggest that theophylline clearance is decreased during serologically confirmed upper respiratory tract infections (Leeder and Kearns 1997).

Elkahwaji et al. (1999) found that in patients with metastatic disease in the liver, high doses of IL-2 decreased the total P450 and monooxygenase activity, specifically the activity of 1A2, 2C, 2E1, and 3A4.

Oncostatin M is a cytokine in the IL-6 receptor family. Although oncostatin M is not used in clinical oncology, this cytokine's presence in disease states makes it notable. Guillen et al. (1998) compared the effects of oncostatin M with those of interferon-γ and IL-6. The activity of 1A2 was noted to be significantly reduced by all three cytokines but most strongly by oncostatin M. Similar reductions in activity of 2A6, 2B6, and 3A4 were noted with exposure to oncostatin M.

■ SUMMARY

This chapter serves as a basic reference for physicians treating patients with multiple pharmacological agents that are involved in the complicated metabolism of the P450 enzymes. The drugs used in the field of clinical oncology are often toxic. Although there is ample evidence to suggest that the P450 enzymes play a role in antineoplastic drug metabolism, there is a clear need for further investigation of the drugs' metabolism. There is also a need for further exploration of genetic polymorphisms and their clinical importance in pharmacokinetics.

■ REFERENCES

Adedoyin A, Stiff DD, Smith DC, et al: All-*trans*-retinoic acid modulation of drug-metabolizing enzyme activities: investigation with selective metabolic drug probes. Cancer Chemother Pharmacol 41:133–139, 1998

Ando Y, Shimizu T, Nakamure K, et al: Potent and non-specific inhibition of cytochrome P450 by JM216, a new oral platinum agent. Br J Cancer 18:1170–1174, 1998

Bagniewski PG, Reid JM, Ames MM, et al: Increased etoposide clearance in patients with glioma may be associated with concurrent glucocorticoid or anticonvulsant treatment (abstract). Proceedings of the Annual Meeting of the American Association for Cancer Research 37:A1224, 1996

Balis FM: Pharmacokinetic drug interactions of commonly used anticancer drugs. Clin Pharmacokinet 11:223–235, 1986

Berkery R, Cleri LB, Skarin AT: Oncology: Pocket Guide to Chemotherapy. St. Louis, MO, Mosby Year–Book, 1997

Berthou F, Dreano Y, Belloc C, et al: Involvement of cytochrome P450 3A family in the major metabolic pathways of toremifene in human liver microsomes. Biochem Pharmacol 47:1883–1895, 1994

Bohnenstengel F, Hofmann U, Eichelbaum M, et al: Characterization of the cytochrome P450 involved in side-chain oxidation of cyclophosphamide in humans. Eur J Clin Pharmacol 51:297–301, 1996

Chan JD: Pharmacokinetic drug interactions of vinca alkaloids: summary of case reports. Pharmacotherapy 18:1304–1307, 1998

Chang P, Riggs CE, Scheerer MT, et al: Combination chemotherapy with adriamycin and streptozotocin, II: clinicopharmacologic correlation of augmented adriamycin toxicity caused by streptozotocin. Clin Pharmacol Ther 20:611–616, 1976

Chang TK, Yu L, Maurel P, et al: Enhanced cyclophosphamide and ifosfamide activation in primary human hepatocyte cultures: response to cytochrome P-450 inducers and autoinduction by oxazaphosphorines. Cancer Res 57:1946–1954, 1997

Chladek J, Martinkova J, Sispera L: An in vitro study on methotrexate hydroxylation in rat and human liver. Physiol Res 46:371–379, 1997

Chen L, Yu LJ, Waxman DJ: Potentiation of cytochrome P450/cyclophosphamide-based cancer gene therapy by coexpression of the P450 reductase gene. Cancer Res 57:4830–4837, 1997

Christians U, Schmidt G, Bader A, et al: Identification of drugs inhibiting the in-vitro metabolism of tacrolimus by human liver microsomes. Br J Clin Pharmacol 41:187–190, 1996

Clarke SJ, Rivory LP: Clinical pharmacokinetics of docetaxel. Clin Pharmacokinet 36:99–114, 1999

Crewe HK, Ellis SW, Lennard MS, at al: Variable contribution of cytochromes P450 2D6, 2C8 and 3A4 to the 4-hydroxylation of tamoxifen by human liver microsomes. Biochem Pharmacol 53:171–178, 1997

Debruyne FJ, Murray R, Fradet Y, et al: Liarozole—a novel treatment approach for advanced prostate cancer: results of a large randomized trial versus cyproterone acetate. Liarozole Study Group. Urology 52:72–81, 1998

Dehal SS, Kupfer D: CYP2D6 catalyzes tamoxifen 4-hydroxylation in human liver. Cancer Res 57:3402–3406, 1997

Desai PB, Duan JZ, Zhu YW, et al: Human liver microsomal metabolism of paclitaxel and drug interactions. Eur J Drug Metab Pharmacokinet 23:417–424, 1998

Dorr RT: Interferon-alpha in malignant and viral diseases: a review. Drugs 45:177–211, 1993

Elkahwaji J, Robin MA, Berson A, et al: Decrease in hepatic cytochrome P450 after interleukin-2 immunotherapy. Biochem Pharmacol 57:951–954, 1999

Gorski JC, Hall SD, Becker P, et al: In-vivo effects of interleukin-10 on human cytochrome P450 activity. Clin Pharmacol Ther 67:32–43, 2000

Goss PE: Pre-clinical and clinical review of vorozole, a new third generation aromatase inhibitor. Breast Cancer Res Treat 49 (suppl 1):S59–S65; discussion S73–S7, 1998

Goss PE, Oza A, Blackstein M, et al: A Phase II study of liarozole fumarate in postmenopausal women with metastatic breast cancer (abstract). Proceedings of the Annual Meeting of the American Society of Clinical Oncology 15:A156, 1996

Grimm SW, Dyroff MC: Inhibition of human drug metabolizing cytochromes P450 by anastrozole, a potent and selective inhibitor of aromatase. Drug Metab Dispos 25:598–601, 1997

Guillen MI, Donato MT, Jover R, et al: Oncostatin M down-regulates basal and induced cytochromes P450 in human hepatocytes. J Pharmacol Exp Ther 285:127–134, 1998

Han IS, Choi JH: Highly specific cytochrome P450-like enzymes for all-*trans*-retinoic acid in T47D human breast cancer cells. J Clin Endocrinol Metab 81:2069–2075, 1996

Harris JW, Rahman A, Kim BR, et al: Metabolism of taxol by human hepatic microsomes and liver slices: participation of P450 3A4 and an unknown P450 enzyme. Cancer Res 54:4026–4035, 1994

Hassan M, Oberg G, Bjorkholm M, et al: Influence of prophylactic anticonvulsant therapy on high-dose busulfan kinetics. Cancer Chemother Pharmacol 33:181–186, 1993

Hill DL, Kirk MC, Struck RF: Microsomal metabolism of nitrosoureas. Cancer Res 35:296–301, 1975

196

Jamis-Dow CA, Pearl ML, Watkins PB, et al: Predicting drug interactions in-vivo from experiments in-vitro: human studies with paclitaxel and ketoconazole. Am J Clin Oncol 20:592–599, 1997

Kajita J, Kuwabara T, Kobayashi H, et al: CYP3A4 is mainly responsible for the metabolism of a new vinca alkaloid, vinorelbine, in human liver microsomes. Drug Metab Dispos 28:1121–1127, 2000

Kim SY, Han IS, Yu HK, et al: The induction of P450-mediated oxidation of all-*trans* retinoic acid by retinoids in head and neck squamous cell carcinoma cell lines. Metabolism 47:955–958, 1998

Kivisto KT, Villikka K, Nyman L, et al: Tamoxifen and toremifene concentrations in plasma are greatly decreased by rifampin. Clin Pharmacol Ther 64:648–654, 1998

Krekels MD, Verhoeven A, van Dun J, et al: Induction of the oxidative catabolism of retinoid acid in MCF–7 cells. Br J Cancer 75:1098–1104, 1997

Kusuhara H, Suzuki H, Sugiyama Y: The role of P-glycoprotein in the liver. Nippon Rinsho 55:1069–1076, 1997

Lee JS, Newman RA, Lippman SM, et al: Phase I evaluation of all-*trans* retinoic acid with and without ketoconazole in adults with solid tumors. J Clin Oncol 13:1501–1508, 1995

Leeder JS, Kearns GL: Pharmacogenetics in pediatrics: implications for practice. Pediatr Clin North Am 44:55–77, 1997

Levin VA, Stearns J, Byrd A, et al: The effect of phenobarbital pretreatment on the antitumor activity of 1,3-bis(2-chloroethyl)-1-nitrosourea (BCNU), 1-(2-chloroethyl)-3-cyclohexyl-1-nitrosourea (CCNU) and 1-(2-chloroethyl)-3-(2,6-dioxo-3-piperidyl-1-nitrosourea (PCNU), and on the plasma pharmacokinetics and biotransformation of BCNU. J Pharmacol Exp Ther 208:1–6, 1979

Liddle C, Goodwin BJ, George J, et al: Separate and interactive regulation of cytochrome P450 3A4 by triiodothyronine, dexamethasone, and growth hormone in cultured hepatocytes. J Clin Endocrinol Metab 83:2411–2416, 1998

May-Manke A, Kroemer H, Hempel G, et al: Investigation of the major human hepatic cytochrome P450 involved in 4-hydroxylation and *N*-dechloroethylation of trofosfamide. Cancer Chemother Pharmacol 44:327–334, 1999

McLeod HL: Clinically significant drug-drug interactions in oncology. Br J Clin Pharmacol 45:539–544, 1998

Monsarrat B, Chatelut E, Alvinerie P, et al: Modification of paclitaxel metabolism by drug induction of cytochrome P450A4 in a cancer patient (abstract). Proceedings of the Annual Meeting of the American Association for Cancer Research 38:A31, 1997

Neuman MG, Cameron RG, Haber JA, et al: Inducers of cytochrome P450 2E1 enhance methotrexate-induced hepatotoxicity. Clin Biochem 32:519–536, 1999

Philip PA, Ali-Sadat S, Doehmer J, et al: Use of V79 cells with stably transfected cytochrome P450 cDNAs in studying the metabolism and effects of cytotoxic drugs. Cancer Chemother Pharmacol 43:59–67, 1999

Rahman A, Korzekwa KR, Grogan J, et al: Selective biotransformation of Taxol to 6-alpha-hydroxytaxol by human cytochrome P450 2C8. Cancer Res 54:5543–5546, 1994

Reid JM, Kuffel MJ, Miller JK, et al: Metabolic activation of dacarbazine by human cytochromes P450: the role of CYP1A1, CYP1A2, and CYP2E1. Clin Cancer Res 5:2192–2197, 1999

Relling MV, Nemec J, Schuetz EG, et al: O-Demethylation of epipodophyllotoxins is catalyzed by human cytochrome P450 3A4. Mol Pharmacol 45:352–358, 1994

Royer I, Monsarrat B, Sonnier M, et al: Metabolism of docetaxel by human cytochromes P450: interactions with paclitaxel and other antineoplastic drugs. Cancer Res 56:58–65, 1996

Santner SJ, Rosen H, Osawa Y, et al: Additive effects of aminoglutethimide, testololactone, and 4-hydroxyandrostenedione as inhibitors of aromatase. J Steroid Biochem 20:1239–1242, 1984

Santos A, Zanetta S, Cresteil T, et al: Metabolism of irinotecan (CPT-11) by CYP3A4 and CYP3A5 in humans. Clin Cancer Res 6:2012–2020, 2000

Schwartz EL, Hallam S, Gallagher RE, et al: Inhibition of all-*trans*-retinoic acid metabolism by fluconazole in-vitro and in patients with acute promyelocytic leukemia. Biochem Pharmacol 50:923–928, 1995

Seidmon EJ, Trump DL, Kreis W, et al: Phase I/II dose-escalation study of liarozole in patients with stage D, hormone-refractory carcinoma. Ann Surg Oncol 2:550–556, 1995

Shet MS, McPhaul M, Fisher CW, et al: Metabolism of the antiandrogenic drug (flutamide) by human CYP1A2. Drug Metab Dispos 25:1298–1303, 1997

Shou M, Martinet M, Korzekwa KR, et al: Role of human cytochrome P450 3A4 and 3A5 in the metabolism of Taxotere and its derivatives: enzyme specificity, interindividual distribution and metabolic contribution in human liver. Pharmacogenetics 8:391–401, 1998

Simpson ER, Zhao Y, Agarwal VR, et al: Aromatase expression in health and disease. Recent Prog Horm Res 52:185–214, 1997

Sonneveld E, van den Brink CE, van der Leede BM, et al: Human retinoic acid (RA) 4-hydroxylase (CYP26) is highly specific for all-*trans*-RA and can be induced through RA receptors in human breast and colon carcinoma cells. Cell Growth Differ 9:629–637, 1998

van Meerten E, Verweij J, Schellens JH: Antineoplastic agents: drug interactions of clinical significance. Drug Saf 12:168–182, 1995

Villikka K, Kivisto KT, Maenpaa H, et al: Cytochrome P450-inducing antiepileptics increase the clearance of vincristine in patients with brain tumors. Clin Pharmacol Ther 66:589–593, 1999

■ CHEMOTHERAPEUTIC AGENTS METABOLIZED AT P450 ENZYMES

3A4	2B1[1]	2C9	2C19	1A2	1A1, 2E1
Busulfan	Cyclophosphamide	Carmustine	Cyclophosphamide	Dacarbazine	Dacarbazine
Cyclophosphamide[2]	Ifosfamide	Paclitaxel	Ifosfamide	Flutamide	
Daunorubicin					
Dexamethasone					
Docetaxel					
Doxorubicin					
Etoposide					
Ifosfamide					
Ondansetron					
Paclitaxel					
Tamoxifen					
Teniposide					
Tetrahydrocannabinol					
Toremifene					
Vinblastine					
Vincristine					
Vindesine					
Vinorelbine					

[1]Very minor human P450 pathway.
[2]N-dealkylation to a neurotoxic agent, chloroacetaldehyde.

■ CHEMOTHERAPEUTIC AGENTS THAT ARE INHIBITORS OF P450 ENZYMES

3A4	1A2	2C9	2D6
Anastrozole	Anastrozole	Anastrozole	Phenothiazines
?Doxorubicin	Flutamide[1]		
?Paclitaxel			

[1]Flutamide's primary metabolite is a **potent** 1A2 inhibitor.

■ CHEMOTHERAPEUTIC AGENTS THAT ARE INDUCERS OF P450 ENZYMES

3A4	2C9	2E1
?Cisplatin	Cyclophosphamide	Retinoids
Cyclophosphamide	Ifosfamide	
Ifosfamide		

15

SURGERY

This chapter covers a collection of seemingly unrelated topics. To maintain the specialty focus of Part III, we have placed pain control and immunosuppressants together under the surgery umbrella. Gynecology has its own chapter. Surgeons of course also use antibiotics frequently; the reader is referred to Chapter 12 for information on these agents. Anesthetic agents engender many drug interactions, but they are rarely encountered by most physicians and are not included here. In this chapter, we refer to antibiotics regularly, because significant drug interactions occur between pain medications, immunosuppressants, and antibiotics.

> Reminder: In this chapter, only P450-mediated interactions are discussed. Interactions due to displaced protein-binding, alterations in absorption or excretion, and pharmacodynamic interactions are not covered.

■ ANALGESICS

Nonsteroidal Anti-inflammatory Drugs

Nonsteroidal anti-inflammatory drugs (NSAIDs) include diclofenac, indomethacin, piroxicam, ibuprofen, and the like, as well as the newly released cyclooxygenase-2 inhibitors. All NSAIDs are metabolized at 2C9 and also undergo phase II metabolism, particularly glucuronidation. The most potent inhibitors of this enzyme are fluvoxamine, fluconazole, and ritonavir (see Chapter 7). Inhibition of these drugs may lead to worsened side effects and/or gastrointesti-

■ ANALGESICS

Drug	Metabolism	Enzyme(s) inhibited	Enzyme(s) induced
Nonopioid/nonsteroidal drugs			
Cyclooxygenase-2 inhibitors	2C9, phase II	None known	None known
Nonsteroidal anti-inflammatory drugs	2C9, phase II	None known	None known
Opioids			
Alfentanil	3A4	None known	None known
Buprenorphine[1]	Phase II	None known	None known
Codeine	2D6, 3A4	None known	None known
Fentanyl	3A4	None known	None known
Hydrocodone	2D6, 3A4	None known	None known
Methadone	3A4	3A4[b]	None known
Morphine	Phase II	None known	None known
Oxycodone	2D6, 3A4	None known	None known
Remifentanil	Not P450[2]	None known	None known
Sufentanil	3A4	None known	None known
Tramadol	2D6, 3A4	None known	None known

[1] Agonist-antagonist opioid.
[2] Ester hydrolysis.

[a] Potent (bold type).
[b] Moderate.
[c] Mild.

nal toxicity. Effectiveness may be lost when NSAIDs are administered with 2C9 inducers such as rifampin.

Morphine

Oxidation is the primary route of metabolism for most opiates, but morphine undergoes glucuronidation, making this agent the safest choice when drug interactions or hepatic insufficiency are considerations (Tegeder et al. 1999). Codeine is metabolized to morphine by *O*-demethylation at 2D6.

Methadone

Methadone is metabolized at 3A4. When this agent is administered with an inducer of 3A4, opiate withdrawal may occur. Altice et al. (1999) reported on a series of seven human immunodeficiency virus (HIV)–positive patients in a methadone maintenance program who were administered the antiviral nevirapine, a potent inducer of 3A4. The patients developed opiate withdrawal symptoms. There are also reports of methadone withdrawal with coadministration of that drug and rifampin, another potent 3A4 inducer (Holmes 1990; Kreek et al. 1976). Altice and colleagues (1999) suggested that methadone and rifampin may be coadministered if higher doses of methadone are prescribed. Caution is needed if patients discontinue the inducing medication (nevirapine, rifampin, carbamazepine, phenobarbital, phenytoin), because it may take several weeks for the effects of induction to diminish, and opiate toxicity may gradually develop if patients are not simultaneously weaned from opiate therapy. Methadone is also subject to inhibition by potent 3A4 inhibitors such as nefazodone, fluvoxamine, ritonavir, and ketoconazole, all of which may decrease metabolism and increase serum levels of parent (active) methadone. Iribarne et al. (1997) reported in vitro evidence that methadone is an inhibitor at 3A4 as well.

Codeine

Codeine and synthetic codeine drugs (oxycodone, hydrocodone) undergo extensive hepatic metabolism. The parent drugs are poor

analgesics. Much of the parent drug is immediately glucuronidated
and excreted as an inactive compound. *N*-Demethylation at 3A4
produces norcodeine, and *O*-demethylation at 2D6 produces morphine, the most active and effective metabolite. *O*-Demethylation
by 2D6 enzymes occurs in the liver and the brain. The site of local
codeine *O*-demethylation in the brain to morphine may be the major
site of effectiveness (Sindrup and Brosen 1995). *O*-Demethylation
at 2D6 is also affected by a patient's genotype. In poor metabolizers
(PMs), analgesia produced by codeine tends to be less than that produced by opiates not dependent on 2D6 for metabolism. Similarly,
if an extensive metabolizer is given a potent inhibitor of 2D6 such
as fluoxetine, paroxetine, cimetidine, quinidine, or ritonavir, 2D6 is
unavailable or competitively inhibited, preventing codeine's metabolism to morphine (Otton et al. 1993; Persson et al. 1995). In a randomized, double-blind, crossover study involving 10 healthy
volunteers, all extensive (average) metabolizers, who received quinidine with oxycodone, significant inhibition of oxycodone metabolism occurred (Heiskanen et al. 1998). There seemed to be no
adverse effect on psychomotor effects or subjective drug effects of
oxycodone, but the sample was small, and the subjects were not in
pain. Because all selective serotonin reuptake inhibitors are inhibitors of 2D6, and because tricyclic antidepressants (TCAs), in addition to regulating sleep, seem to have a central effect on pain,
administering TCAs to patients with chronic pain makes good
sense. TCAs also have the added benefit of readily available serum
levels, a helpful tool in the setting of polypharmacy.

Tramadol

Tramadol is an analgesic with a low affinity for opioid receptors.
Tramadol is also metabolized at 2D6 from parent drug to an active
metabolite, called M1, and is subject to 2D6's polymorphism. PMs
at 2D6 have little or no response to tramadol. Extensive metabolizers may be "converted" to PMs by potent inhibitors of 2D6 such as
paroxetine (Poulsen et al. 1996).

Summary

NSAIDs are all metabolized at 2C9 and may be affected by potent inhibitors and inducers of that enzyme. The opiate analgesics may be associated with multiple drug interactions, with potentially life-threatening outcomes. Few patients being treated for pain receive opiates alone. Many patients with pain are also prescribed antibiotics perioperatively, given TCAs for depression and pain management, or are HIV positive. Potent inhibitors of 2D6 attenuate the metabolism of codeine to morphine. Patients administered such inhibitors may not achieve adequate analgesia, and patients who are PMs at the 2D6 enzyme will not achieve pain control. Potent inducers of 2D6 may, over a 2- to 3-week period of chronic coadministration, reduce the effectiveness of opiates, unless the dose is increased. If the inducer is discontinued, weaning of the patient from opiate therapy is necessary, to prevent opiate overdose as 2D6 downregulates. Tyndale et al. (1997) suggested that PMs at 2D6 enzyme may be "protected" from becoming opiate dependent. These investigators genotyped patients who did or did not meet criteria for oral opiate dependence. The authors found no PMs among those with opiate dependence but significantly more PMs in the never-dependent group.

■ IMMUNOSUPPRESSANTS

Transplant recipients are given immunosuppressants to prevent organ rejection. In addition to drugs such as cyclosporine and tacrolimus (formerly known as FK-506), most organ transplant recipients are also taking medications for hypertension, diabetes, infectious processes, and pain. Distribution, metabolism, and excretion of drugs may all be altered because of disease and drug interactions. We report here on the immunosuppressants and their P450-mediated interactions. In general, drug interactions that lead to increased levels of immunosuppressants may lead to toxicity with serious effects, such as nephrotoxicity. Drug interactions that decrease serum levels of immunosuppressants may lead to organ rejection.

■ IMMUNOSUPPRESSANTS

Drug	Metabolism site(s)	Enzyme(s) inhibited	Enzyme(s) induced
Cyclosporine	3A4	3A4[b]	None known
Muromonab-CD3 (Orthoclone OKT3)	Not P450	None known	None known
Rapamycin (sirolimus)	3A4	3A4[c]	None known
Tacrolimus (FK 506)	3A4	3A4[b,c]	None known

[a]Potent (bold type).
[b]Moderate.
[c]Mild.

Cyclosporine

There are many reports in the literature on interactions between cyclosporine and other agents. As seen in the table, cyclosporine has the potential to inhibit tacrolimus metabolism. This finding was obtained in human liver microsome studies (Iwasaki et al. 1993). Many drugs *inhibit* cyclosporine metabolism, leading to increased serum levels and potential toxicity. Inhibitors verified in in vivo studies include norfloxacin (McLellan et al. 1995), ketoconazole, fluconazole (Sud et al. 1999), calcium-channel blockers, clarithromycin (Spicer et al. 1997), muromonab-CD3 (Orthoclone OKT3), nefazodone, fluvoxamine, and grapefruit juice. Potential inhibitors include any potent inhibitor of 3A4, such as ritonavir, erythromycin, and other agents listed in the table of inhibitors in Chapter 5. *Induction* of cyclosporine metabolism may lead to transplant failure. Carbamazepine and rifampin have been reported to decrease serum cyclosporine levels, and ticlopidine and troglitazone may also decrease these concentrations (Boissonnat et al. 1997; Cooney et al. 1995; Kaplan et al. 1998). St. John's wort was recently found to be an inducer at 3A4, and two patients suffered acute heart transplant rejection due to coadministration of cyclosporine with St. John's wort (Ruschitzka et al. 2000). There have been other reports of transplant rejection when patients added St. John's wort to their immunosuppressant (cyclosporine) regimen (Barone et al. 2000; Karliova et al. 2000).

Exploitation of the inhibition of cyclosporine metabolism has been attempted. Grapefruit juice was given to healthy volunteers taking cyclosporine, and the effect was hypothesized to be cost saving (Min et al. 1996; Yee et al. 1995). The risks of using grapefruit juice are outlined in Chapter 5. Consistency in juice concentration is a significant factor to consider. The calcium-channel blockers diltiazem and verapamil were found to have cyclosporine-sparing effects (i.e., to inhibit 3A4) as well (Leibbrandt and Day 1992; Sketris et al. 1994). Jones (1997) gave a relatively current review of this topic. The potential risk of toxicity or noncompliance due to increased pill burden and side effects may outweigh the economic benefit of such strategies. Vella and Sayegh (1998) and Wright et al. (1999) presented cases in which nefazodone and fluvoxamine increased serum cyclosporine and creatinine levels. Although lower doses of the expensive cyclosporine were possible, patients were subject to more frequent monitoring and blood sampling, procedures that may be particularly poorly tolerated by depressed or anxious patients. Patients may also experience organ rejection if the inhibiting agent is stopped suddenly, which will rapidly decrease serum cyclosporine concentrations (Moore et al. 1996).

Tacrolimus and Rapamycin

The macrolide immunosuppressants tacrolimus and rapamycin (sirolimus) are metabolized at 3A4 and may have inhibitory effects there as well. These agents have narrow therapeutic windows and are associated with nephrotoxicity and cognitive impairment in overdose. Olyaei et al. (1998) reported that 1 week of nefazodone therapy caused new onset of confusion and visual changes, associated with increased serum creatinine levels, in a stable renal transplant recipient. Vasquez and Pollak (1997) reported that tacrolimus (FK-506) increased cyclosporine levels. Mignat (1997) conducted a broad review of the newer immunosuppressants.

Summary

Potent inhibitors and inducers of 3A4 metabolism may greatly affect immunosuppressants, leading to nephrotoxicity or transplant failure. The addition of a potent inhibitor may make it possible to decrease the dose of an administered immunosuppressant—and thus reduce the cost of immunosuppressant therapy—but the risks of exploitation of the drug interaction may outweigh the benefits. Nefazodone and fluvoxamine have been implicated in interactions with these drugs. Serial monitoring of serum immunosuppressant and creatinine levels is recommended by most authors.

209

■ REFERENCES

Altice FL, Friedland GH, Cooney EL: Nevirapine induced opiate withdrawal among injection drug users with HIV infection receiving methadone. AIDS 13:957–962, 1999

Barone GW, Gurley BJ, Ketel BL, et al: Drug interaction between St. John's wort and cyclosporine. Ann Pharmacother 34:1013–1016, 2000

Boissonnat P, de Lorgeril M, Perroux V, et al: A drug interaction study between ticlopidine and cyclosporin in heart transplant recipients. Eur J Clin Pharmacol 53:39–45, 1997

Cooney GF, Mochon M, Kaiser B, et al: Effects of carbamazepine on cyclosporine metabolism in pediatric renal transplant recipients. Pharmacotherapy 15:353–356, 1995

Feierman DE, Lasker JM: Metabolism of fentanyl, a synthetic opioid analgesic, by human liver microsomes: role of CYP3A4. Drug Metab Dispos 24:932–939, 1996

Heiskanen T, Olkkola KT, Kalso E: Effects of blocking CYP2D6 on the pharmacokinetics and pharmacodynamics of oxycodone. Clin Pharmacol Ther 64:603–611, 1998

Holmes VF: Rifampin-induced methadone withdrawal in AIDS (letter). J Clin Psychopharmacol 10:44304, 1990

Iribarne C, Dreano Y, Bardou LG, et al: Interaction of methadone with substrates of human hepatic cytochrome P450 3A4. Toxicology 117:13–23, 1997

Iwasaki K, Matsuda H, Nagase K, et al: Effects of twenty-three drugs on the metabolism of FK506 by human liver microsomes. Research Communications in Chemical Pathology and Pharmacology 82:209–216, 1993

Jones TE: The use of other drugs to allow a lower dosage of cyclosporin to be used: therapeutic and pharmacoeconomic considerations. Clin Pharmacokinet 32:357–367, 1997

Kaplan B, Friedman G, Jacobs M, et al: Potential interaction of troglitazone and cyclosporine. Transplantation 65:1399–1400, 1998

Karliova M, Treichel U, Malago M, et al: Interaction of *Hypericum perforatum* (St. John's wort) with cyclosporin A metabolism in a patient after liver transplantation. J Hepatol 33:853–855, 2000

Kharasch ED, Rusel M, Mautz D, et al: The role of cytochrome P450 3A4 in alfentanil clearance: implications for interindividual variability in disposition and perioperative drug interactions. Anesthesiology 87:36–50, 1997

210

Kreek MJ, Garfield JW, Gutjahr CL, et al: Rifampin-induced methadone withdrawal. N Engl J Med 294:1104–1106, 1976

Leibbrandt DM, Day RO: Cyclosporin and calcium channel blockers: an exploitable drug interaction? Med J Aust 157:296–297, 1992

McLellan RA, Drobitch RK, McLellan H, et al: Norfloxacin interferes with cyclosporine disposition in pediatric patients undergoing renal transplantation. Clin Pharmacol Ther 58:322–327, 1995

Mignat C: Clinically significant drug interactions with new immunosuppressive agents. Drug Saf 16:267–278, 1997

Min DI, Ku YM, Perry PJ, et al: Effect of grapefruit juice on cyclosporine pharmacokinetics in renal transplant patients. Transplantation 62:123–125, 1996

Moore LW, Alloway RR, Vera SR, et al: Clinical observations of metabolic changes occurring in renal transplant recipients receiving ketoconazole. Transplantation 61:537–541, 1996

Olyaei AJ, deMattos AM, Norman DJ, et al: Interaction between tacrolimus and nefazodone in a stable renal transplant recipient. Pharmacotherapy 18:1356–1359, 1998

Otton SV, Wu D, Joffe RT, et al: Inhibition by fluoxetine of cytochrome P450 2D6 activity. Clin Pharmacol Ther 53:401–409, 1993

Persson K, Sjostrom S, Sigurdardottir I, et al: Patient-controlled analgesia (PCA) with codeine for postoperative pain relief in ten extensive metabolisers and one poor metaboliser of dextromethorphan. Br J Clin Pharmacol 39:182–186, 1995

Poulsen L, Arendt-Nielsen L, Brosen K, et al: The hypoalgesic effect of tramadol in relation to CYP2D6. Clin Pharmacol Ther 60:636–644, 1996

Ruschitzka F, Meier PJ, Turina M, et al: Acute heart transplant rejection due to Saint John's wort. Lancet 355:548–549, 2000

Sindrup SH, Brosen K: The pharmacogenetics of codeine hypoalgesia. Pharmacogenetics 5:335–346, 1995

Sketris IS, Methot ME, Nicol D, et al: Effect of calcium-channel blockers on cyclosporine clearance and use in renal transplant patients. Ann Pharmacother 28:1227–1231, 1994

Spicer ST, Liddle C, Chapman JR, et al: The mechanism of cyclosporine toxicity induced by clarithromycin. Br J Clin Pharmacol 43:194–196, 1997

Sud K, Singh B, Krishna VS, et al: Unpredictable cyclosporin-fluconazole interaction in renal transplant recipients. Nephrol Dial Transplant 14:1698–1703, 1999

Tegeder I, Lotsch J, Geisslinger G: Pharmacokinetics of opioids in liver disease. Clin Pharmacokinet 37:17–40, 1999

Tyndale RF, Droll KP, Sellers EM: Genetically deficient CYP2D6 metabolism provides protection against oral opiate dependence. Pharmacogenetics 7:375–379, 1997

Vasquez EM, Pollak R: OKT3 therapy increases cyclosporine blood levels. Clin Transpl 11:38–41, 1997

Vella JP, Sayegh MH: Interactions between cyclosporine and newer antidepressant medications. Am J Kidney Dis 31:320–323, 1998

Wright DH, Lake KD, Bruhn PS, et al: Nefazodone and cyclosporine drug-drug interaction. J Heart Lung Transplant 18:913–915, 1999

Yee GC, Stanley DL, Pessa LJ, et al: Effect of grapefruit juice on blood cyclosporin concentration. Lancet 345:955–956, 1995

APPENDIX A

GUIDELINES

■ GUIDELINES FOR PRESCRIBING IN A POLYPHARMACY ENVIRONMENT

Given the modern polypharmacy environment, a clinician may feel hindered in making prescribing decisions, being wary of untoward drug interactions. The use of multiple physicians and pharmacies by patients increases the risk of insufficient clinical coordination of complicated medication regimens. Some basic principles can help guide clinicians and prevent the occurrence of most P450-mediated drug interactions. The following is a list of five basic principles for the clinician. If at all clinically possible:

1. Avoid prescribing medications that either significantly inhibit or significantly induce P450 enzymes.
2. Prescribe medications that are eliminated by multiple pathways (phase I metabolism, phase II metabolism, and/or renal excretion).

Principles 1 and 2 should be weighed concurrently. By following the first principle, a clinician can avoid potential trouble. The serum levels of medications a patient is already taking will not be altered appreciably by the newly introduced medication, and if the patient is later prescribed a new medication by another physician, the prescribing clinician can feel relatively confident that potential drug interactions are less likely.

Similarly, if a clinician follows Principle 2 by prescribing a medication that is eliminated by multiple pathways, future drugs that may be introduced—drugs with the potential of inhibiting or inducing one or two P450 enzymes—will not cause as much of a problem with the original drug. In addition, phenotypic variability may be less of an issue; if the patient lacks full activity of one enzyme, other enzymes will help clear the drug.

3. Prescribe medications that do not have serious consequences if their metabolisms are prolonged either because of concomitant use of a substrate inhibitor or because the patient being treated is a phenotypic poor metabolizer (PM).

Some psychotropic drugs have narrow margins of safety. Pimozide, clozapine, tricyclic antidepressants, many typical antipsychotics, and some antiseizure medications may have serious untoward effects if their metabolisms are significantly prolonged by substrate inhibitors or because of phenotypic variability. Some of these effects are severe cardiac toxicity, seizures, extreme sedation, and extrapyramidal symptoms.

4. Use serum drug level monitoring often when you are concerned about potential P450-mediated interactions.

Although it is not necessary to obtain serum drug levels at all times, drug level monitoring can often be of great assistance when multiple drugs are being administered. Some examples of the practical use of serum drug levels are given in the study cases in Part II.

5. Remind patients to tell you when other physicians prescribe medications for them.

Educating patients about the possibilities of drug interactions will often reduce the risk of such interactions. A prescribing clinician can keep up with possible interactions by asking patients to contact him or her any time a new medication has been prescribed by another clinician.

Some antidepressants and antipsychotics that generally meet the requirements of the first three principles are given in the table below. Although none of the drugs listed are devoid of all potential P450-mediated interactions, this table provides a starting point for choosing agents wisely. We are not endorsing any medication in the table over others with regard to clinical efficacy. More detailed profiles of medications that may be prescribed by psychiatrists, such as antiepileptic agents, are found elsewhere in this book.

There are two other important issues to consider when making prescribing decisions:

1. Metabolism by P450 enzymes does not always inactivate compounds. Some drugs are pro-drugs and are activated by enzymatic action to active or more active compounds. Codeine, tramadol, and some alkylating agents are examples of such agents. Additionally, some drugs, such as bupropion, haloperidol, fluoxetine, and risperidone, are metabolized to equally effective pharmacologically active metabolites.

2. Typically, the older the drug, particularly if the drug was released in the United States before 1990, the less is known about its metabolism by P450 enzymes. Older drug information on drug-drug interactions is often based on case reports, whereas newer drugs have been better profiled by the manufacturers to enhance their approval by the Food and Drug Administration in the United States. Much of this change occurred after unexpected interactions associated with fluoxetine and with nonsedating antihistamines were reported in the 1980s and 1990s.

■ GUIDELINES FOR ASSESSING AND MANAGING DRUG INTERACTIONS

Polypharmacy cannot be avoided. It is important to remain watchful and to understand the steps for identification and management of drug interactions should they arise. A useful algorithm for attending to drug interactions is found below.

PSYCHOTROPICS WITH FEW P450 INTERACTIONS

Drug	Significant inhibition or induction of P450 (Principle 1)	Metabolism, metabolism site(s), and/or elimination (Principle 2)	Good margin of safety at high serum levels (Principle 3)
Antidepressants			
Bupropion[1]	?2B6 induction, ?2D6 inhibition[8]	2B6, 3A4, others	No[1]
Citalopram	None	3A4, 2C19, renal excretion	Yes
Mirtazapine	None	2D6, 3A4, 1A2, phase II conjugation	Yes
Reboxetine	None	3A4, renal excretion	Yes
Sertraline	Inhibits 2D6 at high doses[2]	2D6, 3A4, 2C9, 2C19, 2B6	Yes
Venlafaxine	None	2D6, 3A4, 2C9, 2C19	Yes
Antipsychotics			
Haloperidol	?3A4 inhibition, 2D6 inhibition[3]	3A4, phase II conjugation	Yes
Molindone	None	?Phase I and II conjugation[4]	
Olanzapine	None	1A2,[5] 2D6, monoamine oxidase, phase II conjugation	Yes
Quetiapine	None	3A4,[6] ?others	Yes
Risperidone	None	2D6,[7] 3A4	Yes

■ PSYCHOTROPICS WITH FEW P450 INTERACTIONS *(continued)*

[1]Bupropion is metabolized to several pharmacologically active metabolites. This drug also appears to induce a minor P450 enzyme, 2B6. High serum levels of bupropion can lead to seizures.

[2]Clinically significant inhibition at doses exceeding 150 mg/day.

[3]Haloperidol has active metabolites. Haloperidol and its metabolites may inhibit 3A4 and 2D6, but not potently.

[4]Molindone's metabolism is not well described in the literature.

[5]Metabolized in multiple ways, but induction of 1A2 has been shown to decrease serum olanzapine levels.

[6]Metabolized mainly by 3A4; other pathways are minor.

[7]Metabolized by 2D6 to an active metabolite.

[8]In vitro data, unpublished.

■ ALGORITHM FOR ASSESSING AND MANAGING DRUG INTERACTIONS

1. Identify interaction

Consult pertinent resources: Resources may include literature identified through *MEDLINE* or other citation databases, drug interactions textbooks or newsletters, commercial drug interaction software programs, or abstracts from conferences. Important information may be obtained from researchers or the manufacturer directly.

Anticipate or predict likely interactions: On the basis of the pharmacology and pharmacokinetics of the suspected medications, would you anticipate a potential interaction? (For example, are the drugs metabolized by the same subset of P450 enzymes? Do they possess enzyme-inhibiting or -inducing properties? Is drug absorption pH dependent or susceptible to cation binding?)

2. Verify existence of interaction

In the literature

How was the interaction described? Was it observed retrospectively, in a study of a single case, in an vitro study, preclinical testing, or a controlled pharmacokinetic human study? In healthy volunteers or a target patient population?

Can the data be applied to your patient population? Was the study population similar to your own? What were the doses and duration of the agent used? Did the subjects have coexisting disease states? Were the subjects taking concomitant medications?

In a clinical situation

What is the time course of the interaction? How long will it take for the interaction to develop? What clinical consequences do you expect to see? Has the interaction already occurred?

Do the clinical signs and symptoms support your assumptions?

Is the objective evidence, such as drug concentrations, available?

Have other potentiating factors been ruled out?

3. Assess clinical significance of interaction

Do the agents involved have a narrow therapeutic index? Are the drugs associated with dose-related efficacy or toxicity?

Is there risk of therapeutic failure or of development of resistance?

4. Evaluate available therapeutic alternatives

Space doses: Can doses be spaced in a practical and/or convenient way for the patient?

Increase dose: Is increasing the dose affordable? Are appropriate dosage forms available?

Decrease dose: Are appropriate dosage forms available?

Discontinue one drug: What are the therapeutic consequences of temporarily or permanently discontinuing one agent?

Change agent: What are the comparative efficacy, adverse effects, cost, availability, compliance issues, and drug interactions associated with a new agent?

Add another agent to counteract effect of interaction: What are the comparative efficacy, adverse effects, cost, availability, compliance issues, and drug interactions associated with a new agent?

Take no action: In certain situations (e.g., when the likelihood of an interaction's occurring is low or when the clinical impact of a potential interaction would be minor or insignificant), the practitioner may want to maintain the patient's current regimen and monitor the patient's condition. Should evidence of a clinically significant interaction be detected, one of the above-mentioned management options may then be considered.

Source. Modified from Tseng AL, Foisy MM: "Management of Drug Interactions in Patients With HIV." Annals of Pharmacotherapy 31:1040–1058, 1997. Used with permission.

220

■ REFERENCES

Callaghan JT, Bergstrom RF, Ptak LR, et al: Olanzapine: pharmacokinetic and pharmacodynamic profile. Clin Pharmacokinet 37:177–193, 1999

Dostert P, Benedetti MS, Poggesi I: Review of the pharmacokinetics and metabolism of reboxetine, a selective noradrenaline reuptake inhibitor. Eur Neuropsychopharmacol 7 (suppl 1):S23–S35, 1997

Fang J, Bourin M, Baker GB: Metabolism of risperidone to 9-hydroxyrisperidone by human cytochromes P450 2D6 and 3A4. Naunyn Schmiedebergs Arch Pharmacol 359:147–151, 1999

Kobayashi K, Ishizuka T, Shimada N, et al: Sertraline N-demethylation is catalyzed by multiple isoforms of human cytochrome P-450 in vitro. Drug Metab Dispos 27:763–766, 1999

Kudo S, Ishizaki T: Pharmacokinetics of haloperidol: an update. Clin Pharmacokinet 37:435–456, 1999

Owen JR, Nemeroff CB: New antidepressants and the cytochrome P450 system: focus on venlafaxine, nefazodone, and mirtazapine. Depress Anxiety 7 (suppl 1):24–32, 1998

Pellizzoni C, Poggesi I, Jorgensen NP, et al: Pharmacokinetics of reboxetine in healthy volunteers: single against repeated oral doses and lack of enzymatic alterations. Biopharm Drug Dispos 17:623–633, 1996

Prior TI, Chue PS, Tibbo P, et al: Drug metabolism and atypical antipsychotics. Eur Neuropsychopharmacol 9:301–309, 1999

Rochat B, Amey M, Gillet M, et al: Identification of three cytochrome P450 enzymes involved in N-demethylation of citalopram enantiomers in human liver microsomes. Pharmacogenetics 7:1–10, 1997

Rotinger S, Bourin M, Akimoto Y, et al: Metabolism of some "second"- and "fourth"-generation antidepressants: iprindole, viloxazine, bupropion, mianserin, maprotiline, trazodone, nefazodone, and venlafaxine. Cell Mol Neurobiol 19:427–442, 1999

Scordo MG, Spina E, Facciola G, et al: Cytochrome P450 2D6 genotype and steady state plasma levels of risperidone and 9-hydroxyrisperidone. Psychopharmacology (Berl) 147:300–305, 1999

Shen WW: The metabolism of atypical antipsychotic drugs: an update. Ann Clin Psychiatry 11:145–158, 1999

Tseng AL, Foisy MM: Management of drug interactions in patients with HIV. Ann Pharmacother 31:1040–1058, 1997

APPENDIX B

HOW TO RETRIEVE AND REVIEW THE LITERATURE

We believe it is important to help readers update this Concise Guide and maintain provider-specific lists themselves. Keeping abreast of the literature may seem daunting, but as providers in the setting of polypharmacy, physicians must do so.

■ SEARCHING THE INTERNET

The Internet is the most powerful, speedy, and all-encompassing way to keep up. How to interface with the Internet is changing daily. Many journals now provide "citation managers" that alert on-line subscribers when topics in which subscribers are interested are cited. Many of these services carry subscription fees.

Web browsers and Web sites are also evolving. Currently, our favorite search engines are *Internet Grateful Med* (www.igm.nlm.nih.gov) and *PubMed* (www.ncbi.nlm.nih.gov/PubMed), in which literature searches tap directly into *MEDLINE*. We have found that the best MeSH terms to use to find literature on P450-mediated drug interactions are *pharmacokinetics, drug interaction, cytochrome,* and the names of the drugs being investigated. We search for articles published from 1985 on and in English, broadening the search by extending the year span and accepting publications in other languages only when several initial tries are fruitless or when we are researching an older drug. We restrict our searches to reports on human studies, because animal studies of the

P450 system are often not translatable to humans or are too preliminary to be useful clinically.

A "great" search, one that is broad enough in scope without being too large for adequate review, should provide the searcher with 20–35 titles. If a searcher retrieves 5–10 and they are exactly what was sought, that result is exceptional and a time-saver. We start with all of the aforementioned MeSH terms, and if not enough titles are retrieved, we eliminate a term at a time, typically dropping *cytochrome* first, because few older reports include this word in the title or abstract. Expanding the range of years searched is necessary in the case of some older drugs, such as phenytoin, phenobarbital, and many of the oncology agents. It should be noted that literature published before 1980 does not directly reflect an understanding of the P450 system, and the searcher may be left making a few leaps and assumptions. In summary, we like to perform a narrow search first. Beginning with a search that is too broad means "wading" through many titles, usually more than 35. Reading through titles and abstracts that may not be needed takes time.

Physicians' Online (www.po.com or www.pol.net) is a Web site with a particularly good drug-interaction tool, the Drug Therapy Monitoring System by Medi-Scan, that feeds directly into *PubMed*. *Physicians' Online* also provides a brief review of the interaction literature and lists all interactions, not just P450-mediated interactions. There are some lapses in the provided data, however, particularly in terms of potential or predictable drug interactions. The best interactive table of drug interactions to date is Dave Flockhart's Drug Table at www.drug-interactions.com. This table is monitored by the Georgetown University Department of Pharmacology, is updated fairly often, and has hyperlinks to literature sources via *PubMed*. The table is restricted to P450-mediated interactions yet is quite complete. A more detailed review of these two sites is found in the spring 2000 issue of *Psychosomatics* (Armstrong and Cozza 2000). Another site, not interactive but more broad than the Physicians' Desk Reference site (www.PDR.net), is Clinical Pharmacology 2000 at Gold Standard Multimedia (www.imc.gsm.com).

■ CRITICALLY REVIEWING THE LITERATURE

Case Reports

Individual cases are often the first clue to a potential drug interaction and were particularly so in the days before human liver microsome studies. Although controls are not involved and confounding variables exist, cases have great merit, especially if they occur with enough frequency to lead to further study, as occurred with terfenadine. A strong case report includes information on pre- and post-administration serum levels of drug, with corresponding clinical effects. Too often, serum levels are missing from case reports. We find it helpful to routinely monitor serum levels of drugs with toxic metabolites or narrow therapeutic windows, especially before administering a new drug with potential interactions, and to obtain another level (at the appropriate time) if a drug interaction is suspected. These data greatly strengthen a case report's credibility. Presentation of a finding of a serum level exceeding clinical standards after administration of a second drug, associated with a significant clinical event, is also common in a strong case report. Monahan et al. (1990) and Katial et al. (1998) have written excellent case reports.

Reports of In Vitro Studies

In the United States, drugs must now be tested for P450-mediated interactions in the laboratory. This testing is done with human liver microsome studies, which permit thorough evaluation of the metabolisms of drugs at the level of the hepatocyte and determine which enzymes will be studied and probed in healthy and patient volunteers. Human liver samples are centrifuged and microsomes are then incubated with the cofactors and enzymes needed for reactions to complete, as well as with test drugs or probe drugs. After completion of the reactions, high-performance liquid chromatography is used for detection of drug or metabolite concentrations. Human liver microsome studies sometimes provide data that do not translate to clinical populations. This lack of clinical correlation is multifactorial and includes differences in culture concentrations and conditions compared with in vivo conditions. Numerous drugs can be tested by these methods, quickly and without impact on volunteers. Zhao et al. (1999) conducted an excellent human liver microsome study.

Reports of In Vivo Studies

Studies involving human volunteers are the gold standard. Studies involving healthy volunteers are usually small ($n = 8–15$), randomized, placebo-controlled studies, sometimes crossover in design. These studies are helpful in determining drug interactions predicted by in vitro studies. The small size of these studies, the frequent use of the single-dose design, and the use of healthy volunteers may limit their generalizability to the general population. Studies involving actual patients, whose ages, diseases, and drug histories vary widely, are some of the strongest studies, particularly if confounding variables are well controlled. Drug concentration, area under the curve (AUC), and maximal drug concentration (C_{max}) are typically measured in these studies. When these parameters as well as pharmacodynamic effect (e.g., psychomotor effects in studies of hypnotics) are studied, the clinical information gleaned can be very helpful. Villikka et al. (1997) conducted an in vivo study with pharmacodynamic correlation. Hesslinger et al. (1999) studied potential drug interactions in psychiatrically ill patients receiving multiple agents.

Review Articles

Review articles are necessary compilations of primary research reports. Reviews allow the sorting and evaluating of research necessary to understand a topic as a whole. These articles help introduce readers to an area of research and provide another viewpoint. A drawback of most reviews is the loss of specific data or of finer arguments and points within individual reports. Many reviews cover only a few drugs or a portion of the P450 system, so several reviews are necessary to compile a full picture. We recommend that reviews be used as guideposts in making clinical decisions. We postpone making final clinical decisions in critical cases until we have examined some of the more specific reports cited by the reviewers themselves or found in our own literature searches.

An excellent introduction to the P450 system was written by Jefferson (1996). Tseng and Foisy (1997) provided tables and text, clearly and with good references, to guide the reader through a complicated area of medicine.

Epidemiological Reports

Population studies help guide the need for drug-interaction research. Jankel and Fitterman (1993) and Hamilton et al. (1998) provided the big-picture reasoning for drug-interaction study. Jankel and co-workers (1993) found that 3% of hospitalizations each year are due to drug-drug interactions. Hamilton and colleagues (1998) confirmed that use of azole antifungals and rifamycins increases the risk of hospitalization because of these drugs' significant P450-mediated drug interactions.

Manufacturer Package Inserts

Manufacturers are important sources of information about their products. The Physicians' Desk Reference (2001) contains the texts of the package inserts of all drugs marketed in the United States. Most of the newer drugs have discrete sections in the manufacturer's insert pertaining to their P450-mediated interactions. We have on many occasions called a manufacturer to obtain postmarketing or not-yet published information about its drugs. Discussions with manufacturers' doctorate-level professionals are generally rewarding and informational.

Summary

A thorough review of the literature concerning a particular drug interaction usually involves reading the package insert and then a few review articles, followed by taking a more focused look at in vitro and in vivo data. All of these research tools are necessary to develop a full understanding of the data available on any drug interaction. Because there are no perfect sources, a compilation similar to this Concise Guide is what each provider will develop about his or her own frequently prescribed drugs.

■ REFERENCES

Armstrong SC, Cozza KL: Consultation-liaison drug-drug interaction update. Psychosomatics 41:155–156, 2000

Hamilton RA, Briceland LL, Andritz MH: Frequency of hospitalization after exposure to known drug-drug interactions in a Medicaid population. Pharmacotherapy 18:1112–1120, 1998

Hesslinger B, Normann C, Langosch JM, et al: Effects of carbamazepine and valproate on haloperidol plasma levels and on psychopathologic outcome in schizophrenic patients. J Clin Psychopharmacol 19:310–315, 1999

Jankel CA, Fitterman LK: Epidemiology of drug-drug interactions as a cause of hospital admissions. Drug Saf 9:51–55, 1993

Jefferson JW, Greist JH: Brussels sprouts and psychopharmacology: understanding the cytochrome P450 enzyme system. Psychiatr Clin North Am 3:205–222, 1996

Katial RK, Stelzle RC, Bonner MW, et al: A drug interaction between zafirlukast and theophylline. Arch Intern Med 158:1713–1715, 1998

Monahan BP, Ferguson CL, Killeavy ES, et al: Torsades de pointes occurring in association with terfenadine use. JAMA 264:2788–2790, 1990

Physicians' Desk Reference, 55th Edition. Montvale, NJ, Medical Economics, 2001

Tseng AL, Foisy MM: Management of drug interactions in patients with HIV. Ann Pharmacother 31:1040–1058, 1997

Villikka K, Kivisto KT, Luurila H, et al: Rifampin reduces plasma concentrations and effects of zolpidem. Clin Pharmacol Ther 62:629–634, 1997

Zhao XJ, Koyama E, Ishizaki T: An in vitro study on the metabolism and possible drug interactions of rokitamycin, a macrolide antibiotic, using human liver microsomes. Drug Metab Dispos 27:776–785, 1999

INDEX

*Page numbers printed in **boldface** type refer to tables or figures.*

    induction by, 148
    inhibition by, 146
        CYP3A4, 48, **66,** 118, 146
Antihistamines, 115–119, **117**
    CYP3A4 inhibition of, 116–118
    metabolism of, 20, 49–50, **63**
Antimalarials, **63**
Antimetabolites, 182–183
    fluorouracil, 183
    methotrexate, 182–183
Antimycobacterials/antitubercular
        agents, 150–153, **151**
    isoniazid, 152, 153
    rifamycins, 150–152
        drug interactions with,
            152–153
        induction by, 150
        inhibition by, 150
        interaction with CYP3A4
            inhibitors, 150
Antineoplastic drugs, 179–192.
        See also specific drugs
    alkylating agents, 180–182
        busulfan, 180
        carmustine, 182
        cyclophosphamide, 181
        ifosfamide, 181
        lomustine, 182
        streptozocin, 182
        trofosfamide, 181–182
    antiandrogens and antiestrogens,
            187–190
        aminoglutethimide, 187–188
        anastrozole, 188
        flutamide, 188

        liarozole, 188–189
        tamoxifen, 189
        toremifene, 189
        vorozole, 190
    antimetabolites, 182–183
        fluorouracil, 183
        methotrexate, 182–183
    antitumor antibiotics, 187
        doxorubicin, 187
    combinations of, 180
    drug interactions with, 179
        azole antifungals, 149
    genetic variability and, 31
    induction by, **200**
    inhibition by, **200**
    metabolism at P450 enzymes,
            63, 199
    miscellaneous agents, 190–192
        cisplatin and other platinum
            agents, 190
        dacarbazine, 190
        retinoids, 190–191
        steroids, 192
    pharmacokinetics in pediatric
            patients, 179–180
    taxanes, 183–185
        docetaxel, 183–184
        paclitaxel, 184–185
    topoisomerase inhibitors,
            186–187
        etoposide, 186
        irinotecan, 186–187
        teniposide, 186
    vinca alkaloids, 185–186
        vincristine, 185
        vinorelbine, 185–186

232

236